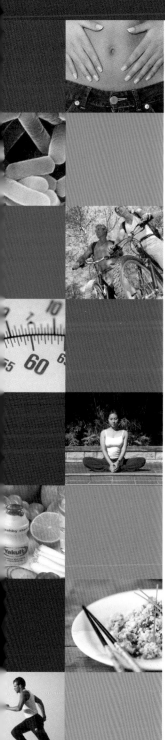

GW00391480

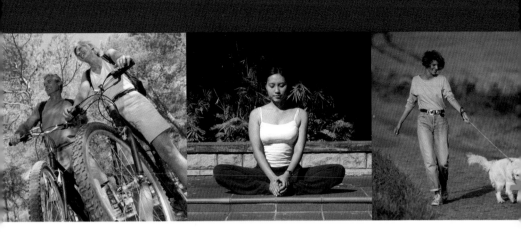

Introduction

Almost all diets focus on weight-loss, food types and calorie content. The Inside Out Diet is different. The Inside Out Diet focuses on the gut.

Statistics show that more than a third of the population claim to have problems with their digestive system. Doctors are diagnosing more people each year with Irritable Bowel Syndrome (IBS) and colitis, and bowel cancer is the second biggest cancer killer in the UK. Even on a less serious level, various aspects of today's hectic lifestyles can upset the health of our gut. Common culprits include inactivity, antibiotics, stress, too much alcohol, a poor diet, smoking, dehydration, overseas travel and lack of sleep.

Meanwhile, the natural ageing process, illnesses, infections or food poisoning, can also play havoc with our digestive system. And when our digestive system is unhappy, it generally lets us know by providing us with unpleasant symptoms.

Yet despite all this, many people are unaware about how important it is to keep the digestive system healthy – or what they should do to take care of it.

That's where The Inside Out Diet can come to the rescue. It's designed to help relieve digestive health problems such as bloating and discomfort, constipation and diarrhoea. But it's not just a diet for 'people with tummy troubles'. The Inside Out Diet has also been devised to prevent digestive problems from occurring in the first place. This is great news because keeping our digestive system healthy may have many other knock-on health benefits in the body such as boosting our energy levels, immunity and mood. And that's not all. Changing our lifestyles to boost the health of our digestive system may also help to protect us from major health problems like heart disease, strokes, high blood pressure, diabetes and certain cancers.

Let's get one thing straight. The Inside Out Diet is not a weight loss plan. Nevertheless, many people may find they lose weight when they follow the diet and lifestyle advice.

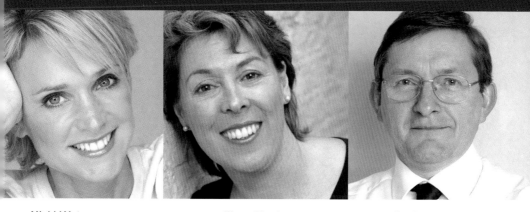

Nicki Waterman   *Fiona Hunter*   *Dr Anthony Leeds*

Better still, The Inside Out Diet is suitable for most adults at anytime – the basic principles can be followed throughout life to keep us healthy and free from disease. However, it's particularly useful at certain times: just before going on holiday or travelling overseas to prepare the digestive system for different foods and a change in lifestyle; during times of stress; or following a course of antibiotics. It also becomes increasingly relevant as people get older, when like everything else, the digestive system starts to show the signs of ageing and begins to slow down. Those who have a medical condition, are pregnant or breastfeeding should consult their doctor before starting a diet.

The Inside Out Diet is designed to help you keep your digestive system – and the rest of your body – as healthy as possible. By taking care of our insides, most people will be healthier, have more energy and look better – as well as possibly losing those excess pounds! Your digestive system is constantly talking to you. Isn't it about time you started to listen?

Here's what The Inside Out Diet may do for you
- boost immunity and fight infection
- give you more energy
- prevent constipation and other tummy troubles
- boost your overall health
- keep your heart healthy
- stop you feeling hungry in between meals
- help you manage your weight

But in order to fully appreciate the daily principles of The Inside Out Diet, it is important that you have some understanding about your digestive system and what can happen when things go wrong.

How the digestive system works

The main function of the digestive system is to take in and process food in order to provide the body with energy (calories) and nutrients. The gut also handles some substances made in the body such as cholesterol and bile salts, and provides an environment for the growth of 'friendly' bacteria needed for good health.

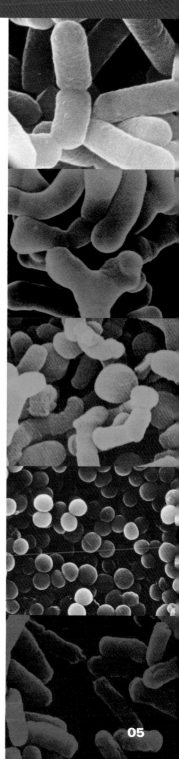

A healthy digestive system generally doesn't cause problems, with the result that most of us don't even think about what's happening to our insides. We may sometimes hear bubbling, gurgling sounds or wind coming up (belching) or going down (flatulence). But in fact, these are only tiny parts of the constant conversation that our digestive system has with other parts of our body, particularly our brain.

Our digestive system is a bit like a miniature factory. Basic materials go in at one end... they're processed... the flow rate is controlled... products are created and diverted to one side... other things are added... yet more products are diverted to the side... and finally a residue passes out at the end. While a factory has pumps to push things forward, our digestive system has waves of muscular movement. While a factory has detectors to check flow rates, our digestive system has hormone messengers and nerve signals to determine the movement of these muscles.

But just like a factory, if the starting material or part of the equipment isn't quite right, the entire production chain is affected and can potentially break down. For example, if our starting material (food) doesn't contain enough fibre, this means our production line has to work overtime to pass the waste out of the body and may sometimes give up for a while (constipation). The good news is it's relatively easy to fix this problem – simply by adding more fibre to our diet.

Bugs in the system

Believe it or not, there are more bacteria in your colon than there are humans on this planet! And just as on this planet, there's competition for space to live. Just as local conditions affect people's preferences for somewhere to live, the local conditions of the large intestine determine the types of bacteria that will grow. Like people, bacteria directly affect their environment: while some bacteria have minimal effect, 'harmful' bacteria may damage their environment and increase the risk of infection, whereas 'good' bacteria (such as those found in Yakult) help keep the environment healthy, often improving digestion and making certain vitamins. The key is to get the right balance of 'good' and 'bad' bacteria in the intestines (or gut). For more information on how to do this see p13.

Here's the lowdown on the different parts of the digestive system and how they work

1 The mouth

Seeing and smelling food starts the digestive process by increasing the flow of saliva in the mouth. Biting and chewing breaks food up and mixes it with saliva, which contains starch-splitting enzymes. The tongue then pushes the chewed food to the back of the mouth, where it's swallowed.

2 The gullet (oesophagus)

Once swallowed, food enters the gullet – a muscular pipe that pushes food from the mouth to the stomach in about six seconds.

3 The stomach

The stomach stores food for anything between just a few minutes and five hours. During this time, the food is mixed with acid. This not only helps digest protein but also kills many bacteria, thus stopping them from entering the gut alive, helping to prevent infections. Only alcohol is absorbed from the stomach into the blood; that's why alcohol can affect you so quickly. Once digestion in the stomach is complete, the ring of muscle at the bottom of the stomach relaxes and allows small quantities of food to pass into the small intestine.

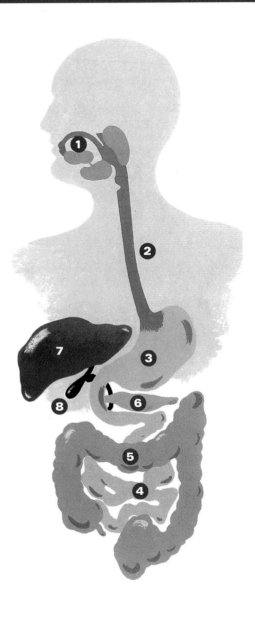

4 The small intestine (duodenum, jejunum and ileum)

The small intestine is about six metres long. It's where most of the digestion of fat, carbohydrate and protein takes place with the help of enzymes released by the pancreas and the intestine itself and bile, which helps to digest fat. The small intestine has a vast surface area to ensure nutrients are absorbed quickly and thoroughly.

5 The large intestine (colon and rectum)

When most of the nutrients have been absorbed, the remaining residue passes into the large intestine, which is home to over four hundred different types of 'good', 'bad' and 'indifferent' bacteria. Some of these bacteria ferment undigested fibre and starch. Then water is removed and absorbed back into the body to create semi-solid stools (faeces). The rectum stores the faeces until it's convenient to expel it from the body via the anal canal – a muscular tube.

6 The pancreas

While not strictly part of the digestive system, the pancreas is essential to digestion. This gland secretes an alkaline juice (which neutralises the acid from the stomach) and enzymes that break down protein, fat and carbohydrates. Some cells of the pancreas also secrete hormones like insulin, which help control blood sugar.

7 The liver

The liver is the chemical factory and warehouse of the body. It receives nutrients from the gut via the blood and metabolises these in many different ways. It also stores some nutrients such as vitamin B12 and vitamin A and makes bile, which is secreted down a tube called the bile duct into the gall bladder.

8 The gall bladder

The gall bladder concentrates bile and squeezes it into the small intestine, where it helps to digest fat.

CHAPTER 02

What happens when things go wrong?

The digestive system can go wrong in many different ways, but it usually sends out some signals to tell you things aren't right. Abdominal pain, changes in bowel habit, nausea or vomiting are all tell-tale signs that something is wrong.

You should see your practice nurse or doctor for advice if...

- Your bowel habit has changed within the last two to three months and you've not changed your diet, been travelling or started taking medication
- You've seen blood in your stools – new red blood, or black stools containing digested blood
- You have persistent, unexplained abdominal pain or discomfort
- You have lost 2kg (4lb) in weight recently for no obvious reason
- You have lost your appetite and/or frequently feel sick for no obvious reason
- You are frequently constipated and simple treatments such as a high-fibre diet, more fluids, more exercise and over-the-counter laxatives haven't worked
- You frequently open your bowels more than three times a day or if your stools are often loose or watery
- You frequently get a lot of unexplained wind, bloating or abdominal distension

How can I tell if I'm constipated? It's a good indication that you are constipated if you...

- Open your bowels less than three times a week
- Strain to open your bowels more than one time in four
- Pass hard or pellet-like stools more than one time in four

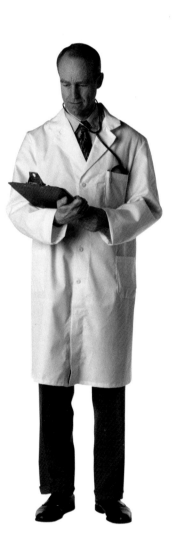

View your poo!

You might not like doing it, but looking into the toilet pan can help you identify the health of your digestive system. The chart below identifies the most common type of stools. Type 1 has spent the longest time in the colon; stools at this end of the scale are hard to pass and often require a lot of straining. In contrast, type 7 has spent the least time in the colon; stools at this end of the scale often need to be passed urgently to prevent an accident. The ideal stools are types 3 and 4, especially type 4; these are the easiest to pass, the least likely to leave you with the feeling that something is left behind and they indicate optimal functioning of the digestive system.

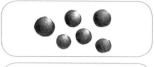

Type 1
Separate hard lumps like nuts (difficult to pass)

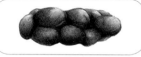

Type 2
Sausage shaped but lumpy

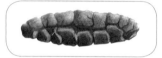

Type 3
Like a sausage but with cracks on surface

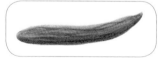

Type 4
Like a sausage or snake, smooth and soft

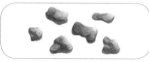

Type 5
Soft blobs with clear-cut edges (passed easily)

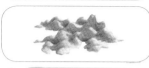

Type 6
Fluffy pieces with ragged edges, a mushy stool

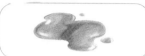

Type 7
Watery, no solid pieces (entirely liquid)

Courtesy of The Bristol Scale (ref: BMJ, 1990)

Now we've seen what can go wrong with the digestive system, it's time to discover how we can keep it in perfect working order.

Eating for a healthy digestive system

Unsurprisingly, eating a healthy, balanced diet is the easiest way to help keep our digestive system - and every other part of our body - in tip top shape. And the easiest way to achieve this is to eat plenty of different foods from four main groups and limit the amount we eat from a smaller fifth group. Ultimately, we should eat more fruit, vegetables, starchy, fibre-rich foods and fresh products, and fewer fatty, sugary, salty and processed foods. Here's the lowdown...

Bread, other cereals and potatoes

Foods in this group include bread, rice, pasta, noodles, breakfast cereals, yams, oats and grains. These foods provide energy, small amounts of protein, vitamins, minerals and fibre. Healthy eating guidelines suggest eating these foods at each meal and having them as snacks if we're hungry. Whenever possible, wholegrain varieties such as wholemeal bread, wholegrain breakfast cereals, brown rice and pasta should be chosen. Aim for 3 or more servings a day.

> **One serving equals...**
> - 2 slices bread in a sandwich or with a meal
> - a tennis ball sized serving of pasta, potato, rice, noodles or couscous
> - a bowl of porridge
> - a handful of breakfast cereal

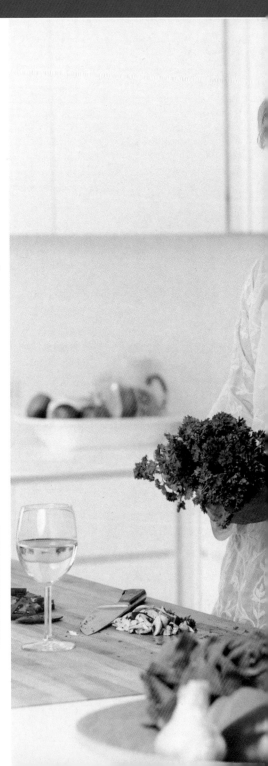

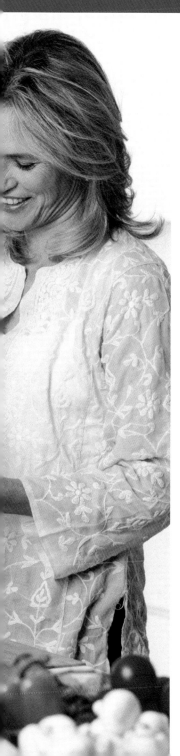

Fruit and vegetables

Foods in this group include fresh, frozen, canned and dried fruits and vegetables as well as juices. Fruit and vegetables provide a range of vitamins and minerals, fibre and naturally occurring plant chemicals called phytochemicals. The World Cancer Research Fund estimates that a diet rich in a variety of fruit and vegetables could prevent 20% of all cancers. We should all eat at least 5 servings of fruit and vegetables a day – and because no one fruit or vegetable provides all the vitamins or phytochemicals we need to stay healthy, it's important to eat a variety.

One serving equals...
- a small glass (150ml) unsweetened fruit juice or vegetable juice – but this only counts as one serving a day no matter how much you consume
- 1 apple, orange, peach, pear
- 2 kiwi fruits, plums, satsuma or fresh apricots
- 1 slice of melon or pineapple
- 1 cup of strawberries, raspberries or grapes
- 1tbsp dried fruits/raisins
- 3tbsp fruit salad or cooked or canned fruit
- 3tbsp cooked vegetables
- a 'breakfast-sized' bowl of salad

Milk and dairy foods

Foods in this group include milk, yogurt, cheese and fromage frais. Dairy products are an important source of calcium, essential for strong bones and teeth. Many women, especially teenage girls, fail to eat enough calcium to meet their daily needs, putting themselves at risk of osteoporosis (weakened bones) in later life, which can increase the risk of fracture. Dairy foods also provide protein, vitamin A, phosphorus, vitamin D and vitamin B2. Foods in this group can be high in fat, particularly saturated fat so choose reduced-fat and low-fat alternatives such as skimmed and semi-skimmed milk. We should aim to eat 2–3 servings a day from this group.

One serving equals...
- 1 glass (200ml) of milk
- a small pot (around 150g) of yogurt or fromage frais
- a small matchbox-sized (30g) piece of cheese

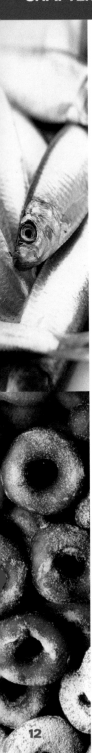

Meat, fish and alternatives

Foods in this group include meat, fish, poultry, eggs, beans, nuts and seeds. These foods provide protein, essential for the growth and repair of the cells and the production of enzymes, antibodies and hormones. Foods in this group also provide several important vitamins and minerals. We should aim to eat 2 servings from this group a day. If you choose meat, make sure it's lean and trim away any visible fat before cooking. It's also important to eat at least 2 servings of fish a week – one of which should be an oil-rich variety such as salmon, mackerel or fresh tuna. Oil-rich fish are packed with omega-3 fatty acids, which can reduce cholesterol levels in the blood and make the blood less sticky and less likely to clot, therefore helping to reduce the risk of heart disease and strokes.

One serving equals...
- a piece of meat, chicken or fish the size of a deck of cards
- 1-2 eggs
- 3 heaped tablespoons of beans
- a small handful of nuts or seeds

Limit the amount of food eaten from this group:

Fatty and sugary foods

Small amounts of fat are necessary in our diet to provide us with essential fatty acids and to allow the absorption of fat-soluble vitamins, but most of us eat far more than is good for us. Many fatty foods in this group are also rich in saturates, which raise blood cholesterol and increase the risk of heart disease. Meanwhile, sugar provides 'empty' calories – calories that provide nothing else in the way of protein, fibre, vitamins or minerals.

These foods should only be eaten in small amounts...
- oils, spreading fats, mayonnaise, cream
- cakes, biscuits, pastries, puddings
- crisps, chips, salty savoury snacks
- sugar, preserves and confectionery

Healthy eating made easy

Food group	How much each day?
bread, other cereals and potatoes	at least 3 servings
fruit and vegetables	at least 5 servings
milk and dairy foods	2-3 servings
meat, fish and alternatives	2 servings
fatty and sugary foods	limit these foods

Digesting the facts

While a healthy, balanced diet is essential for all round good health, there are also some specific things you can eat to help to keep the digestive system in perfect working order.

Boost those friendly bacteria - Probiotics

Probiotics are live bacteria that improve the balance of good and bad bacteria in the gut. The most common probiotic bacteria are bifidobacteria and lactobacilli – found in products like Yakult. Unlike the live bacteria in ordinary yoghurts, probiotic bacteria survive the acidic conditions of the stomach and pass into the small and large intestines. Once there, these good bacteria compete for the limited space in the gut and in doing so, help to control levels of harmful bacteria. The good bacteria may also help to boost our immune system, protecting us from disease. By changing certain immune responses, probiotics may also help to ease conditions like colitis (inflammation of the large gut). Since movement in the gut is affected by bacteria, conditions caused by excessive movement or spasm (such as Irritable Bowel Syndrome) or slow bowel movement (one cause of constipation) may also be improved by taking probiotics. And in other conditions where the gut flora may be disturbed, such as following the use of antibiotics or after a bout of traveller's diarrhoea, probiotics may help to restore normal function.

Feed those healthy bacteria - Prebiotics

Getting a daily dose of friendly bacteria by having a probiotic drink every day is a great way to look after your gut. However, if you want to do everything possible to keep your digestive system healthy, you should also eat foods which help to stimulate growth of these good bacteria – known as prebiotics.

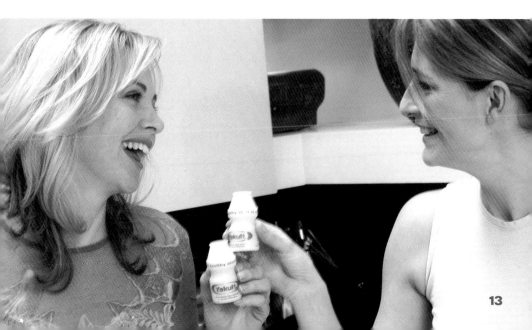

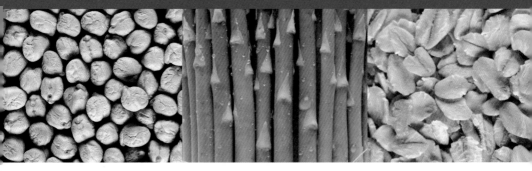

Fortunately, this isn't too hard as good sources of prebiotics include many carbohydrates made from the sugar fructose. These types of carbohydrates occur in the Allium group of plants (onions, garlic, shallots, leeks), and in asparagus, chicory and artichokes, as well as to a lesser extent in beans and pulses (such as chickpeas and lentils) and some cereals, e.g. oats. Inulin, a pure form of fructose that is not digested in the small intestine is also a good food for probiotic bacteria that and is sometimes added to other foods by food manufacturers to boost and enhance probiotic growth.

Quite simply, if you want those good bugs to thrive it is best to include some prebiotic foodstuffs in your daily diet. For some great prebiotic recipes see p32-47.

Fill up on fibre

It's a common known fact that dietary fibre is essential to a good diet, but its actual benefits are not so widely understood. There are two main types of fibre: insoluble and soluble fibre, both with their individual benefits to the digestive system. Foods that contain insoluble fibre can act as a laxative which helps prevent constipation, whilst large amounts of soluble fibre can help reduce blood cholesterol levels and can also help people with diabetes control their blood glucose levels.

Good sources of insoluble fibre include wholegrain cereals and wholemeal bread and beneficial sources of soluble fibre include oats, fruit, vegetables, beans and pulses.

Resistant starch

Resistant starch is a component of starch which is not digested in the small intestine because it is too dry or enclosed within plant cell walls. It contributes to the amount of fermentable carbohydrate that passes undigested to the large bowel. Sources of resistant starch may help achieve a slower release of glucose from the food into the blood stream. Resistant starch can be found in a variety of foods including wholegrains, legumes, pasta, potatoes and bread.

Enjoy meat - but in small amounts

Studies have shown a link between eating large amounts of red meat (particularly processed meat), and colorectal (bowel) cancer.

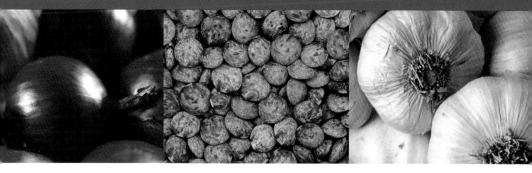

This shouldn't completely put you off red meat as it provides a good source of protein, iron and minerals in the diet. Obesity and lack of exercise are far stronger risk factors for bowel cancer, while eating plenty of fruit and vegetables may well help to lower the risk.

Here are some guidelines for enjoying meat...

- Eat meat as part of a balanced diet that includes plenty of fibre-rich veg, beans and pulses, wholegrain cereals, fruit and vegetables – a good intake of these appears to counteract any increase in risk linked to high intakes of red or processed meat.
- Choose modest portions – aim to eat no more than 140g/5oz of red or processed meat a day.
- Sometimes, swap processed meats like burgers, ham, bacon and sausages for lean red meat.

Healthy wholegrains

For a healthier diet, try switching refined carbs such as white rice, white bread, sugary cereals and white pasta for wholegrain varieties. When grains are refined, for example to make white flour or white rice, the outer bran and germ layers of the grain are stripped away. Sadly, this is where much of the fibre and many of the nutrients and phytochemicals are concentrated. So when these layers are removed during processing, the grain also loses many of its nutrients. While fortification adds certain nutrients back to the refined grain, this doesn't take into account the whole package that Mother Nature provided. It's becoming increasingly clear that it's the natural combination of fibre, nutrients and phytochemicals that gives wholegrains their many health benefits.

Of course, a good intake of wholegrains is particularly good for the gut as they contain more fibre. But a growing body of evidence suggests that people who eat at least three servings of wholegrains each day are also less likely to suffer from heart disease, type 2 diabetes and certain types of cancer. Meanwhile, other research suggests wholegrains may play a role in treating and preventing obesity because they are more filling than their refined counterparts. Indeed, a study of American nurses found that those who ate a diet high in fibre and wholegrains were least likely to be overweight.

CHAPTER 04

A healthy weight for a healthy digestive system

Being overweight or obese affects all aspects of our health and also has an effect on our digestive system. Fat stored around the midriff can put pressure on the stomach - tending to squash food already mixed with stomach acid back up into the gullet. This can cause heartburn and, if left untreated, painful ulceration.

But that's not the only way in which obesity affects our digestive system.

Fibre provides the bulk that helps to speed the passage of waste food through the bowel. The kind of high-fat, high-sugar, low-nutrient diets that often lead to weight gain are usually also low in fibre. A low fibre diet results in harder, more compact stools which take longer to pass through, resulting in constipation. That's why many overweight and obese people have problems with constipation, which can be so easily combated with a few simple dietary changes.

Poor diet and lack of fibre in the digestive system will also increase the risk of developing haemorrhoids (piles) as straining to pass hard dry stools causes an increase in intestinal pressure forcing weakly supported engorged veins out through the back passage.

How do I know if I'm overweight?

Take a look at the Body Mass Index (BMI) chart on p60. Your BMI is a way of finding out if your weight is putting your health at risk. All you need to know is your height and weight.

In addition to your BMI, research shows that fat stored around our middle – sometimes called central obesity – is also far more dangerous to our health than fat that's stored around our bottom and hips. Central obesity is a risk factor for metabolic syndrome – which increases the risk of diabetes and heart disease. A waist measurement greater than 102cm (40in) for men and 88cm (35in) for women means you need to take urgent action to lose weight.

Help... I need to lose weight!

Don't panic – you're not alone. In fact, a massive 65% of men and 56% of women in the UK are overweight or obese and should really be taking action to shift those excess pounds and improve their health. Fortunately, The Inside Out Diet may help you to lose weight.

In the meantime, here are some starting points...

- Set yourself a weight or BMI target – make it realistic though and set yourself a suitable time limit. Remember, you didn't pile on those pounds overnight so you can't expect to lose them overnight either.
- Use the food diary at the back of this book – write down everything you eat.
  Then look at where you can make simple changes to reduce your daily calorie intake. You only need to cut 500 calories a day, to lose 0.5kg (1lb) in a week – and that soon mounts up to a stone!
- Also use the planner to look at some of your lifestyle habits; eg: record how much TV you are watching, how much activity you are getting – you may be surprised that you are not as active as you may think.
- Plan your meals in advance and shop wisely.
- Don't skip meals, especially breakfast – you'll end up overcompensating later in the day.
- Start moving – regular exercise will help to build muscle and burn extra calories. Turn to p48 for more information.

Easy ways to cut calories without even noticing...

- Choose low – and reduced–fat alternatives of your favourite foods
- Go for low – and reduced-fat dairy products
- Choose lean meat and skinless chicken
- Grill, bake, poach, boil, steam or dry roast instead of frying
- Read the label and choose foods with less than 3g fat per 100g or per serving
- Eat filling, wholegrain foods instead of refined foods
- Eat plenty of vegetables and fruit – go for 5 a day
- Keep vegetable and fruit snacks handy so you can nibble on them instead of reaching for chocolates, biscuits or cakes
- Drink sparkling water instead of fizzy drinks
- Drink alcohol in moderation only – alcohol will remove your inhibitions so that you're more likely to drink and eat even more
- Don't eat while you're walking, talking or travelling – concentrating on what you eat will help to slow down the speed at which you eat, so that you recognise feelings of fullness sooner
- Limit fast foods and takeaways – they tend to be high in fat, calories and salt

How your lifestyle can affect your digestive system

Even people who have a healthy diet can experience digestive problems. This is because the balance of bacteria in our gut is affected by a wide variety of everyday factors. Common culprits include stress, lack of sleep, over-indulgence in rich food or alcohol and smoking. Meanwhile, the natural ageing process, as well as illness or food poisoning can also play havoc with our digestive system.

Sleep

Believe it or not, the amount of sleep we get can affect our bowel habits. Just like the rest of our body, our digestive system needs time to relax and recuperate. Unfortunately, many of us don't get enough sleep because we stay up late watching TV – and this often goes hand in hand with late night snacking, which makes our digestive system go to work when it should be resting. Munching in the early hours can mean we're more likely to put on weight – indeed, studies show that insufficient sleep can lead to weight gain – and this puts even more pressure on the digestive system.

Meanwhile, too little sleep can affect our performance at work and make us feel irritable and stressed. And of course, stress can have a major impact on the health of our digestive system.

Finally, going to bed and getting up at regular hours each day can help our digestive system work more effectively and improve the regularity of our bowel habits.

Try some of these tips to ensure a good night's sleep...
- Decide how much time you need to get ready in the morning before leaving for work, then calculate backwards to work out the time you need to be in bed to get a good 7–8 hours sleep.
- Plan your evening meals and snacks so that you don't eat too late – avoid eating a large meal within 2–3 hours of going to bed and avoid foods and drinks that disturb you.
- Prepare for sleep by winding-down for 1–2 hours before you go to bed.
- Make sure your mattress, pillows and bed linen are as comfortable as possible.
- If your partner snores encourage him or her to seek treatment for the condition.

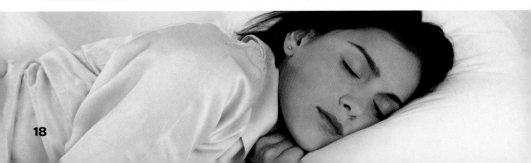

Inactivity and TV

Just like the rest of our body, our digestive system benefits from regular physical activity. When we don't exercise it regularly, it simply becomes sluggish and we may start to feel bloated, windy, lethargic and may experience abdominal pain. The Inside Out Diet contains exercise suggestions to help get you and your digestive system going (see p48). However the problem of inactivity is quite deeply rooted in the habits of modern society and this can be harder to address.

The balance between physical activity and physical inactivity is seriously out of kilter in today's society. For many of us, work is now a relatively sedentary 'activity' that exercises only a limited number of small muscles. Many of us are also so exhausted after working long hours that our 'play-time' is also based around sitting in front of a TV screen – spending more and more of our active hours being inactive. But how can we address this? Again, it is a question of planning – addressing exactly what you are doing now and deciding how to change it. Which is why it is good to look at your 'television history' when trying to make changes in your digestive health:

Ask yourself these questions:
- How much time do you spend on average each day sitting in front of the TV/computer screen/computer game screen?
- Do you eat in front of the TV?
- Could you plan your TV viewing?
- Could you do some physical activity whilst watching (like ironing)?
- Could you bear to be selective and cut out some programmes?

You may be surprised by how much time you are spending sitting in front of the screen per week. There is increasing evidence that the inactivity associated with TV viewing or other screen use may increase risk of being overweight and becoming diabetic. More than about two hours each day may be too much for some people. Keep a simple diary of how much time you spend at your computer screen at work, watching TV at home and any other screen use, then see if there is any scope for reducing this.

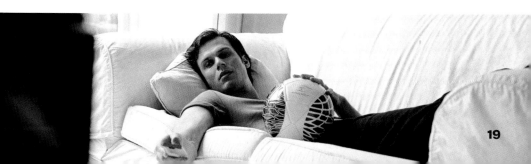

Travel

Going on holiday or taking a trip abroad can play havoc with our digestive system. New research by Yakult reveals a staggering 10 million Brits have had their holidays abroad ruined due to digestive problems. One in five have suffered from gut problems on holiday experiencing either diarrhoea or constipation. A despairing two thirds of these succumb to a digestive health problem every time they travel.

Long periods of inactivity on the plane or by the pool, changes in air cabin pressure, dehydration, and different eating and drinking habits, can all contribute to holiday bloating, constipation or diarrhoea. Although there are obvious precautions you can take once you're abroad – such as avoiding the local tap water and ice, peeling fruit and veg, and skipping food that looks like it's been kept warm for hours – many people don't realise it's possible to take action to help protect their gut before they even set off. By preparing your digestive system in the weeks before your holiday, you can minimise the chances of falling ill once you're there.

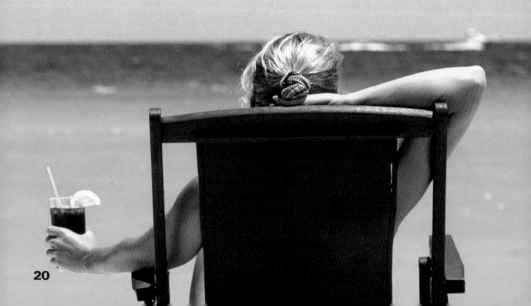

Top tips for boosting your defences against any nasty travel bugs:

- Turn to p26 and start to follow The Inside Out Diet – ensuring that you take a probiotic and several servings of prebiotics every day before you travel
- Remember to start the diet at least two weeks before your trip
- Pack some high-fibre cereal or dried fruits in your suitcase to have for breakfast or as a snack. It's often a challenge to eat enough fibre on holiday and this can soon impact on your digestion.
- Stay hydrated – dehydration is a major cause of gut problems when we're on holiday. It's vital to drink lots of water when you're flying, as air travel can quickly dehydrate you. And don't forget to drink plenty of water once you reach your destination.
- Pack a good diarrhoea and a constipation remedy, just in case you feel unwell – it's easier than trying to find a suitable medicine in a foreign country.
- Move around regularly – if you're travelling on a plane do your leg exercises as described in the flight handbook and if possible take a walk. Once on holiday jump in the water once an hour if you are relaxing by the pool. Long periods of inactivity can make your digestive system sluggish.
- Get your digestive system in tip top shape in the run up to, and during your holiday by following some specific exercises (see p48).

Antibiotics

An estimated 36 million courses of antibiotics are prescribed in the UK each year to help kill bacteria that cause infections. However, as well as killing harmful bacteria, many antibiotics also kill beneficial bacteria that keep our digestive system healthy. In fact, when we take antibiotics, up to 60% of the total amount of bacteria in our gut – both good and bad – can be killed. The result can sometimes be diarrhoea.

Trying to counter the negative effects of antibiotics can be important. To help avoid the unwanted side effects of antibiotics try the following...

- Eat plenty of foods containing prebiotics such as onions, garlic, leeks, asparagus and artichokes. These foods help the friendly bacteria in the digestive system to multiply.
- Have a probiotic drink every day. These drinks contains billions of friendly bacteria to top up good levels of bacteria in the gut.
- Doctors will only prescribe antibiotics if there is a good reason – but do not be afraid to question your doctor if you have any doubts about its effects.

Alcohol

Drinking too much alcohol doesn't just affect the liver. It's toxic to every part of the body, including the brain, the pancreas, the muscles and even our digestive system. Alcohol is at its most concentrated in the stomach – especially when no food is present – and as a result, when consumed in large amounts can cause irritation and inflammation of the stomach lining. This in turn may result in nausea and vomiting.

Alcohol is absorbed from the stomach into the bloodstream. Nevertheless, some alcohol still passes into the small intestine where it limits the ability to process nutrients and vitamins. Continual heavy drinking can result in inflammation of the stomach and it has been linked to cancer of the intestines.

Once alcohol has been absorbed from the stomach and small intestine, it's taken to the liver – the main detox organ in the body – which is then put under tremendous pressure to break it down and remove it from the body.

Most of us know the feeling after a heavy session of drinking… along with a throbbing headache usually comes a dodgy tummy! Alcohol affects our bowel movements as it prevents our small and large intestines from reabsorbing salt and water, resulting in diarrhoea.

In order to avoid the unpleasant side effects of too much alcohol, it's important to drink sensibly and avoid exceeding recommended limits for alcohol. Men should drink no more than four units a day. Women should drink no more than three units a day. It's also important to have at least one alcohol-free day each week.

One unit of alcohol is equivalent to:
- A single (25ml) measure of spirits
- A small (125ml) glass of medium strength wine
- A half pint of ordinary-strength lager, beer or cider

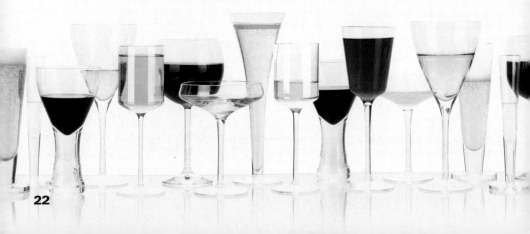

Follow these tips to help you drink sensibly...

- Offer to drive so that you can stick to non-alcoholic drinks all night.
- Start a night out with a couple of non-alcoholic drinks – many people are thirsty when they first arrive at a bar or pub, so quench this thirst with alcohol-free beverages.
- Mix wine with soda or sparkling water.
- Don't drink neat spirits – always add a mixer like orange juice or tonic water.
- Pace yourself and have one non-alcoholic drink after every alcoholic one.
- Don't be afraid to skip rounds and when it's your round buy a non-alcoholic drink for yourself (if friends or colleagues pile on the pressure to keep drinking, tell them it's an alcoholic drink – a lemonade looks just like a gin and tonic!)
- Avoid doubles – and watch out for trendy bars that serve them as the standard. Many pubs now also sell 35ml measures as the standard instead of the more usual 25ml measure. These contain around 1.5 units each.
- Use a spirits measure for drinks at home rather than pouring freely from the bottle.
- Be wary with alcopops – they often don't taste alcoholic so it's easy to drink large amounts. If you like the fruity taste, choose fruit juice mixed with lemonade.
- If you feel under pressure to drink, make up an excuse for sticking to alcohol-free drinks, for example, tell people you are dieting or you're taking antibiotics.
- Don't smoke while drinking – doing the two together greatly increases the risk of mouth cancer.

Smoking

You've heard it hundreds of times before, but smoking is bad for your whole body, including your digestive system.

Smoking is responsible for many changes in the digestive system. It contributes to common disorders such as heartburn and peptic ulcers. Smoking also increases the risk of Crohn's disease and gallstones. Another reason to try and quit is that smoking decreases your liver's ability to handle alcohol, so the two combined are double trouble for the digestive system.

Top Tips:

- To help you quit, set a date for stopping smoking
- Ensure that friends and family know and are supportive
- Throw away anything that you associate with smoking, including ash trays and lighters
- Expect to get withdrawal symptoms and a cough when you first stop
- Avoid situations where you know you'll want to smoke
- Get support – turn to p59 for support organisations who can help you quit.

Stress

Stress is a normal part of life in today's modern society and small amounts may actually be good for us, helping us to perform more effectively. However, problems arise when our lives cause an abnormal amount of stress.

One of the first parts of the body to react to stress is our digestive system.

What's the worst that can happen just before an important job interview or an important exam? A bad bout of diarrhoea? Unfortunately, diarrhoea is a common side effect of stress. This occurs as the adrenalin that's pumping around your body when you're feeling stressed speeds everything up, including the rate at which food is passed through your body.

Meanwhile, it's not just stress itself that can affect our digestive system. Being stressed also means we're more likely to indulge in lifestyle habits that are also bad for our digestive system. Being stressed means we may be more likely to smoke, drink excessive amounts, take less exercise or eat a poor, unbalanced diet. Combined with the effects of adrenaline, stress can have a disastrous affect on our gut.

To avoid unwanted stress, sit down with a pen and paper and work through the following...

- Identify the things that make you feel stressed – see if there is anything you can do to easily eliminate some of these things from your life
- Look at how you react to the things that stress you out – and decide whether your reactions are appropriate.
- Write a list of possible solutions to the things that stress you – for example, could you delegate to other people?
- Find ways to reduce stress – this might be as simple as doing some simple breathing exercises, taking up yoga or meditation, indulging in a weekly massage, or just taking a walk or going for a swim – these really do work.
- You may even want to consider re-evaluating your goals and objectives in life so that you can switch to a low-stress lifestyle.
- Turn to p48 for some stress-busting exercises.

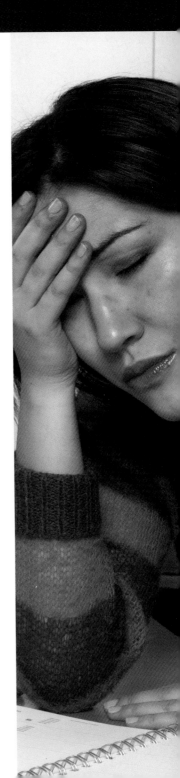

Dehydration

Staying hydrated is essential to the health of your digestive system. The human body needs water to maintain enough blood and other fluids to function properly. As soon as the body begins to lose a substantial amount of water more quickly than it is replaced, the body starts to get dehydrated.

A common effect of dehydration on your digestive system is constipation. Many people become dehydrated without even realising it – this is because thirst is not a good guide to dehydration. To prevent dehydration, aim to drink 6-8 glasses of water a day – more when the weather is warm – and should increase this intake when doing any form of exercise or in a hot climate.

Check list
- Drink at least 6–8 glasses of water a day – in warm weather you'll need to drink more.
- Don't rely on thirst as a sign that you need to take a drink.
- Eat plenty of fruit and vegetables will help increase your fluid intake.
- Take water breaks rather than coffee breaks at regular intervals during the day.
- Keep a bottle of water on your desk at work to remind you to take a drink.
- Drink plenty of water before, during and after taking exercise – especially when the weather is warm.

Getting older

Ageing not only affects the way we look on the outside. As we get older, the bacteria living in our gut also change, tipping more in favour of harmful bacteria. Levels of beneficial bacteria may drop and as we get older our immune systems become weaker. As 80% of the immune system is gut-associated it is important that the gut's beneficial bacteria are maintained to support it.

Meanwhile, several digestive disorders are more common as we get older, making it even more essential to look after our digestive system. In particular, older adults are more likely to develop diverticular disease or suffer with constipation, due to both a slowing in the movement of contents through the large intestine and reduced contractions in the rectum that let us know we need to empty our bowels.

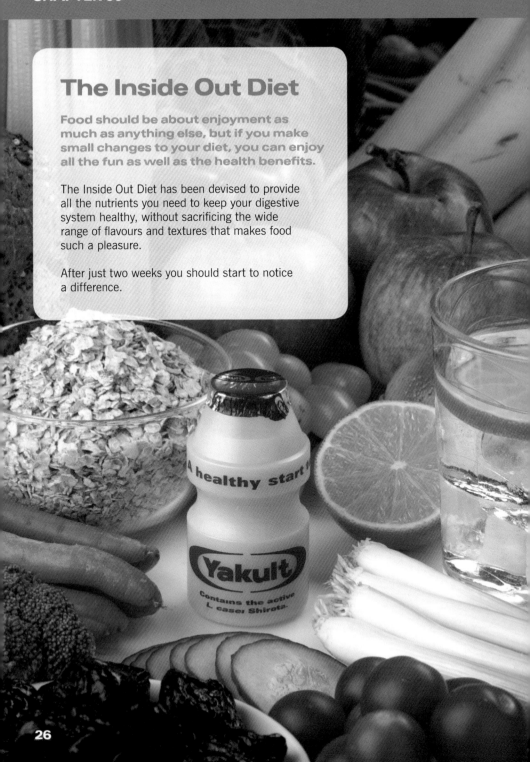

The Inside Out Diet

Food should be about enjoyment as much as anything else, but if you make small changes to your diet, you can enjoy all the fun as well as the health benefits.

The Inside Out Diet has been devised to provide all the nutrients you need to keep your digestive system healthy, without sacrificing the wide range of flavours and textures that makes food such a pleasure.

After just two weeks you should start to notice a difference.

Here's why The Inside Out Diet is so good for your digestive system...

- It contains a daily probiotic drink to boost levels of good bacteria in the gut
- It includes five portions fruit and veg every day – these are packed with vitamins and minerals but also contain good amounts of fibre, needed to keep the digestive system in good health
- It includes three servings of wholegrains every day – such as wholemeal pasta, brown rice, wholegrain cereals, oats and wholemeal bread. Once again these are a great source of fibre
- It includes plenty of prebiotic foods such as onions, leeks, asparagus, oats and bananas to feed those healthy bacteria
- It keeps processed carbohydrates, including sugars, to a minimum
- It's low in saturated fat, but includes plenty of the heart healthy fats found in foods like nuts, olive oil and avocados
- It keeps salt to a minimum

So now you know the basics, it couldn't be easier to follow. Here's what to do...

- Every morning, start your day with a bottle of probiotic drink such as Yakult
- Then simply follow the daily menu plans
- As well as your probiotic drink, meals and snacks, you should also have 300ml of semi-skimmed milk each day for using in tea and coffee, to drink on its own or to combine with fruit to make a smoothie
- You should also serve meals with plenty of vegetable or salads – aim for five servings of fruit and veg each day
- Remember to drink plenty of water – you should have six-eight glasses a day. It's also fine to drink small amounts of tea and coffee, herbal and fruit teas and sugar-free soft drinks
- If you want to speed up weight loss, simply opt for smaller portions, for example, have one slice of bread instead of two

Use the planner at the end of the book not only to record what you have eaten in the day but also what lifestyle decisions you have made – how many hours of TV you have watched, how much physical activity you have undertaken, how much water you have drunk. Then plot your progress and see if you can improve on your results day-by-day following the advice in the guide so far.

Day 1

Start the day	1 probiotic drink
Breakfast	One serving of porridge with prunes and apricots (see p32) and one serving of carrot, apple and kiwi juice (see p33)
Lunch	Chicken and spring onion salad: chop 1 grilled skinless chicken breast and 2 spring onions. Mix with 3tbsp sweetcorn and 1tbsp reduced-fat crème fraiche. Serve with a green salad and 1 wholemeal pitta bread. Plus 1 pear
Dinner	One serving of risotto with peas and asparagus tips (see p40)
Snacks	2 oatcakes with 2tsp peanut butter

Day 2

Start the day	1 probiotic drink
Breakfast	½ pink grapefruit, 2 slices wholegrain toast with 2tsp peanut butter and 1 small glass fresh orange juice
Lunch	Three bean salad: chop ½ small red onion, ½ green and red pepper and 5 cherry tomatoes. Mix with 3tbsp each of red kidney beans, butter beans and chick peas, 6tbsp cooked brown rice and fat-free dressing
Dinner	One serving of steamed salmon with olive oil and vegetables (see p42) served with wholewheat pasta
Snacks	Tzatziki with vegetable crudités. Plus a bowl of blueberries and blackberries

Day 3

Start the day	1 probiotic drink
Breakfast	2tbsp porridge oats mixed with 2tbsp branflakes, 2 chopped dried apricots, 1tbsp raisins and 1tsp sunflower seeds with semi-skimmed milk
Lunch	One serving of tomato, mozzarella and avocado salad (see p37) with a chunk of granary bread
Dinner	Lamb kebabs: chop 100g lean lamb into bite-sized pieces. Mix with 2tbsp tzatziki and leave to marinate for 30 minutes. Thread onto three skewers with ½ chopped red and green pepper and 1 small red onion. Grill until the meat is cooked, brushing with the marinade occasionally. Serve with brown rice, salad and more tzatziki (don't use the marinade)
Snacks	Hot tomato salsa (see p47) with vegetable crudities

Day 4

Start the day	1 probiotic drink
Breakfast	One serving of Swiss muesli with blueberries (see p34)
Lunch	One serving of salad Nicoise (see p38)
Dinner	Roasted Mediterranean vegetables: roast 1 green pepper, 1 red pepper, ½ red onion, 5 cherry tomatoes, 1 sliced courgette and 3 slices aubergine with 2tsp olive oil until soft and brown. Top with 50g sliced reduced-fat mozzarella cheese and allow to melt. Serve with a chunk of granary stick and salad with fat-free dressing
Snacks	2 slices wholegrain toast topped with 1 small mashed banana

Day 5

Start the day	1 probiotic drink
Breakfast	2 slices wholegrain toast with 2tsp low-fat spread and 1 boiled egg. Plus 1 small glass fresh orange juice and 1 kiwi fruit
Lunch	One serving of Mediterranean mixed salad (see p36) with a grilled skinless chicken breast. Plus 1 small pot of low-fat fruit yogurt
Dinner	One serving of prawn and vegetable stir fry (see p44) with wholewheat noodles. Plus 1 kiwi fruit, fresh raspberries and a handful of grapes
Snacks	1 wholemeal pitta with tzatziki

Day 6

Start the day	1 probiotic drink
Breakfast	One serving of strawberry, blueberry, cranberry and red grape juice (see p35). Plus 2 Weetabix with semi-skimmed milk
Lunch	2 slices wholegrain bread filled with ½ small can tuna in water mixed with 2tsp reduced-fat mayonnaise, 3 sliced spring onions and salad. Plus 1 small banana
Dinner	One serving of mango chicken with raisins and walnuts (see p44) with brown rice and salad
Snacks	Bowl of raspberries and blueberries topped with 1 small pot low-fat natural yogurt

Day 7

Start the day	1 probiotic drink
Breakfast	One serving of poached eggs with asparagus (see p34) and 1 orange
Lunch	One serving of watercress, chicory, onion, black grape and alfalfa salad (p36) with 1 wholegrain roll
Dinner	1 small grilled lean rump steak with red onions fried in a little olive oil, small serving wholewheat pasta and salad. Plus 1 kiwi fruit
Snacks	2 oatcakes with low-fat soft cheese

Day 8

Start the day	1 probiotic drink
Breakfast	1 slice wholegrain toast, 2 eggs scrambled with a little semi-skimmed milk and grilled mushrooms. Plus 1 small banana
Lunch	One serving of beetroot, pink grapefruit, chicory and red onion salad (see p37) with 1 grilled skinless chicken breast and a small chunk of granary bread
Dinner	Pasta and vegetables in tomato sauce: steam a selection of vegetables. Mix with cooked wholewheat pasta and ½ jar low-fat tomato sauce. Heat though and serve with 1tsp freshly grated Parmesan cheese and salad with fat-free dressing
Snacks	One serving of cantaloupe melon served with summer fruits (see p35)

Day 9

Start the day	1 probiotic drink
Breakfast	One serving of kiwi, raspberry and blueberry crush (see p35) and 1 slice of wholegrain toast with 1tsp peanut butter
Lunch	One serving of tuna fishcakes (see p39) with 1 wholegrain roll
Dinner	Chicken fajitas: cut 1 skinless chicken breast into bite-sized pieces and fry in 1tsp sunflower oil with a little fajita seasoning. When cooked, add ½ sliced red and green pepper and ½ small sliced red onion. Cook until the veg are brown. Fill 2 small flour tortillas with the chicken and veg and 1tbsp each of tzatziki, salsa and guacamole. Serve with any remaining chicken mixture
Snacks	1 slice wholegrain toast with 1tsp each of low-fat spread and honey and 1 pear

Day 10

Start the day	1 probiotic drink
Breakfast	1 slice wholegrain toast with 1tsp low-fat spread and 2 poached eggs. Plus 1 small glass fresh orange juice and 1 kiwi fruit
Lunch	Avocado dip and pitta bread: mash 1 small avocado with 1 skinned and de-seeded chopped tomato, a little lemon juice, Tabasco to taste and 1 clove crushed garlic. Serve with 1 wholemeal pitta bread and vegetable crudités. Plus 1 pot low-fat fruit yogurt
Dinner	1 grilled trout with new potatoes cooked in their skins and salad with fat-free dressing. Plus one serving of plums in red wine and cranberry juice (see p45)
Snacks	2 slices wholegrain toast with 2tsp peanut butter and 1 small banana

Day 11

Start the day	1 probiotic drink
Breakfast	Bowl fresh fruit salad with 1 pot low-fat fruit yogurt and 2tbsp porridge oats
Lunch	1 wholemeal pitta bread filled with 2 hard boiled eggs, sliced spring onions and cress. Plus 1 apple
Dinner	One serving of taboulleh (see p37) with vegetable kebabs: thread three skewers with a selection of chopped vegetables eg button mushrooms, peppers, courgette, aubergine. Brush with olive oil and grill until cooked through and brown
Snacks	Reduced-fat hummus with 2 rye crispbreads. Plus 1 banana

Day 12

Start the day	1 probiotic drink
Breakfast	6tbsp branflakes with 1tbsp raisins and semi-skimmed milk. Plus 1 banana
Lunch	One serving of any low-fat vegetable soup and 2 slices of wholegrain bread filled with 1 slice lean roast beef, 1 sliced tomato and ½ sliced red onion
Dinner	One serving of stuffed red peppers (see p42) with salad
Snacks	3 rye crispbreads with cottage cheese, sliced red onions and chives. Plus 1 apple

Day 13

Start the day	1 probiotic drink
Breakfast	2 slices wholegrain toast with 1 small can plum tomatoes Plus 1 small banana
Lunch	½ carton fresh carrot and coriander soup with 1 toasted wholegrain bagel topped with 2tsp low-fat spread. Plus 1 orange
Dinner	Creamy salmon pasta: mix 6tbsp cooked wholewheat pasta with steamed broccoli, ½ small can pink salmon and 2tbsp low-fat soft cheese with garlic and herbs. Heat through and serve with salad with fat-free dressing
Snacks	Bowl of strawberries and raspberries

Day 14

Start the day	1 probiotic drink
Breakfast	1 toasted wholegrain bagel with 2tbsp low-fat soft cheese and 1 tomato. Plus 1 small glass of fresh pomegranate juice
Lunch	1 jacket potato with cottage cheese, spring onions, salad and fat-free dressing. Plus 1 apple
Dinner	One serving of duck with prunes (see p41) with brown rice
Snacks	3 oatcakes topped with low-fat soft cheese and slices of red onion

Recipes for a healthy digestive system

If you want to get a little more adventurous in the kitchen then try out some of these fantastic recipes by specialist health recipe developer and food writer Sally van Straten. All of these dishes include digestive-friendly ingredients eg fibre, fruit and veg and wholegrains, as well as prebiotics to help feed your good bacteria!

Breakfasts, juices, smoothies & snacks

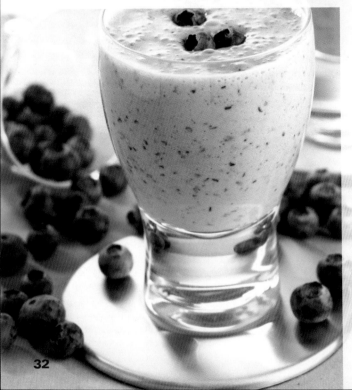

Porridge with prunes & apricots

Porridge makes a great start to the day: protein, B vitamins and slowly-released energy make this the perfect breakfast. Plus don't forget the gut-friendly oats and the antioxidant-rich dried fruit!

Serves 2
Per serving

614 calories	12g fat
7g saturated fat	19g fibre

Ingredients
2 cups semi-skimmed milk
2 cups water
2 cups porridge oats
8 ready-to-eat prunes (snipped)
8 ready-to-eat apricots (snipped)
2tsp brown granulated sugar
Extra milk for drizzling

Method
1. Put the milk and water into a saucepan. Bring to a gentle simmer, stirring occasionally. Add the oats and cook for 5 mins or as directed on the packet.
2. Add the prunes and the apricots to the porridge. Cover and leave for 1 min.
3. Pour into two bowls, sprinkle over the sugar and leave to melt – about 1 min. Serve with extra milk poured on top.

Carrot, apple & kiwi juice

This juice adds an extra nutrient boost to your breakfast.

Serves 4
Per serving
203 calories   <1g fat
0g saturated fat   4g fibre

Ingredients
4 large carrots
  (washed and peeled)
3 good-flavour eating apples
  (washed)
3 kiwi fruit, peeled

Method
1. Put all the ingredients through a juicer, pour into a glass and enjoy.

Strawberry, banana & blueberry smoothie

This contains prebiotic carbohydrate from the banana and live bacteria in the yogurt!

Serves 2
Per serving
194 calories   3g fat
1g saturated fat   2g fibre

Ingredients
1 small banana
6 large strawberries
110g (4oz) blueberries
425ml (15fl oz) live natural yoghurt

Method
1. Slice banana into blender, add half the yoghurt. Switch on, add the rest of the fruit and slowly pour in the rest of the yoghurt.

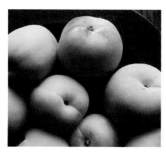

Compote of mixed dried fruits with live yoghurt & flaxseeds

If you're in a hurry in the morning, this is the healthy alternative to stopping on the way to work for coffee and a doughnut. Prepared the night before, it will take you less than five minutes to pour on the yogurt and eat – and it will help get your day off to a flying start.

Serves 2
Per serving
316 calories   13g fat
3g saturated fat   8g fibre

Ingredients
350g (12oz) mixed
  dried fruits eg prunes,
  apricots, mangos, raisins,
  blueberries, apples,
  bananas
2 small live bio yoghurts
2tbsp flax seeds

Method
1. Put the fruit in a large bowl and cover with boiling water. Allow to cool, then put into the fridge overnight.
2. Serve in the morning, with the yogurt poured on top and scattered with flax seeds.

Blueberry, cranberry, blackcurrant & banana cooler

Loads of vitamin C, lots of antioxidants and potassium, energy and prebiotics from the banana.

Serves 2
Per serving
112 calories   <1g fat
0g saturated fat   14g fibre

Ingredients
1 ripe banana
110g (4oz) blueberries
110g (4oz) cranberries,
  defrosted if frozen
110g (4oz) blackcurrants
A handful of ice cubes

Method
1. Whizz all together in a blender.

Orange, pink grapefruit, lime & raspberry juice

This is a real taste treat. You could juice the fruit by hand or in the blender – or simply eat it separately.

Serves 2
Per serving
107 calories   <1g fat
0g saturated fat   8g fibre

Ingredients
2 oranges
1 pink grapefruit
2 limes
110g (4oz) raspberries

Method
1. Simply juice the fruit, pour into glass, add a couple of ice cubes and enjoy.

Blueberry muffins made with prune pureé

It's hard to believe, but this recipe really works. Because prunes are naturally sweet you don't need to add much sugar and prune pureé makes a fabulous substitute for fat!

Makes 8, 2 per serving
Per serving
260 calories   3g fat
1g saturated fat   6g fibre

Ingredients
10 stoneless, ready-to-eat prunes
175g (6oz) half and half plain and wholemeal flour
2tsp baking powder
25g (1oz) caster sugar
1 egg
150ml (5fl oz) semi-skimmed milk
100g (3 and a half oz) blueberries

Method
1. Make a prune pureé by whizzing the prunes in a food processor with a little water. You want them to have the consistency of double cream.
2. Mix together the flours, baking powder and sugar. Beat the egg and mix into the milk and prune pureé. Add to the flour mixture and beat thoroughly. Mix in the blueberries, being careful not to break up the fruit.
3. Divide the mixture between eight deep, greased muffin tins, filling only to just over half their depth. Cook at 200C/400F/gas 6 for 25 mins

Swiss muesli with blueberries

This traditional Alpine start to the day is a far cry from the sawdust texture of cheap muesli. Good muesli is made with oats and lots of raisins, sultanas and other dried fruits so you get instant energy from the fruit sugars, slow-release energy from the oats, calcium and beneficial bugs from the yogurt and a huge amount of vitamin C from the blueberries.

Serves 2
Per serving
404 calories   5g fat
1g saturated fat   4g fibre

Ingredients
2 bowls half filled with good quality, sugar free muesli
About 700ml (1 1/4pints) apple juice
1 small carton plain, full-fat, bio yoghurt
150g (5oz) fresh blueberries

Method
1. Pour the juice onto the muesli – it should almost drown it – then stir in the yoghurt. Cover and leave overnight in the fridge
2. In the morning, wash the blueberries and serve the muesli with the blueberries piled on top.

Poached eggs with asparagus

Definitely not a Monday morning breakfast – unless it's a bank holiday – but a perfect, leisurely weekend brunch. Natural plant chemicals and prebiotics in asparagus make them surprisingly healthy as well as a delicious treat.

Serves 2
Per serving
309 calories   13g fat
4g saturated fat   8g fibre

Ingredients
8 asparagus tips
4 eggs
1tsp vinegar
2 medium sized tomatoes
4 slices wholemeal bread

Method
1. Steam asparagus for 5 minutes
2. Meanwhile, poach the eggs in gently boiling water to which you've added the vinegar and the tomatoes. Don't cook the eggs more than 3-4 mins unless you want them hard.
3. Toast the bread, remove the crusts and cut into triangles. Put one egg on each triangle of toast with one poached tomato. Serve the asparagus tips sprinkled with black pepper and dip asparagus into the runny yolks.

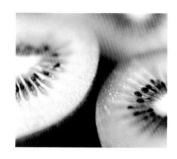

Kiwi, raspberry & blueberry crush

Another vitamin and anti-oxidant rich mixture of these amazingly healthy fruits.

Serves 2
Per serving

179 calories	1g fat
0g saturated fat	2g fibre

Ingredients
2 large kiwi fruit
110g (4oz) mixed raspberries and blueberries
250ml (9fl oz) apple juice
250ml (9fl oz) cranberry juice

Method
1. Whizz together in a blender.

Tea bread with raisins & prunes

The low fat content makes this a treat you can enjoy without a single pang of conscience.

Serves 4
Per serving

649 calories	3g fat
<1g saturated fat	14g fibre

Ingredients
5 Earl Grey tea bags
300ml (10fl oz) boiling water
225g (8oz) prunes (snipped)
1 medium egg (beaten)
225g (8oz) raisins
200g (7oz) brown sugar
250g (9oz) wholemeal self-raising flour

Method
1. Soak the tea bags in the water and leave until cold. Squeeze the tea bags and discard.
2. Mix all the ingredients together and leave for at least six hours.
3. Line a 1.2 litre (2pint) bread tin neatly with greaseproof paper. Spoon in the mixture and bake for 30 mins at 180C/350F/gas 4

Cantaloupe melon filled with summer fruits

As a breakfast, starter, dessert or lunchtime snack, this is refreshing, tasty and unbelievably healthy. The melon provides lots of beta-carotene, for eyes and skin, and all the berries will give you around five times the amount of vitamin C you need for one day. But the real gift from nature in this recipe is its extraordinarily high amount of antioxidants from such a small amount of food.

Serves 2
Per serving

86 calories	<1g fat
0g saturated fat	9g fibre

Ingredients
1 ripe Cantaloupe melon (halved and de-seeded)
175g (6oz) of mixed strawberries, blueberries, blackberries and red currants

Method
1. Heap the soft fruit into the hollows in the melon

Strawberry, blueberry, cranberry & red grape juice

If you haven't got a juicer this mixture makes a terrific smoothie blended with yoghurt. It's a dramatic immune booster because of its high vitamin C content but it's also exceptionally rich in phytochemicals that may help protect against heart disease, some cancers, premature ageing and many infections.

Serves 2
Per serving

89 calories	<1g fat
0g saturated fat	4g fibre

Ingredients
110g (4oz) strawberries
110g (4oz) blueberries
110g (4oz) frozen cranberries, defrosted
110g (4oz) seedless red grapes

Method
1. Put all ingredients into a juicer or add yoghurt and whiz together in a blender.

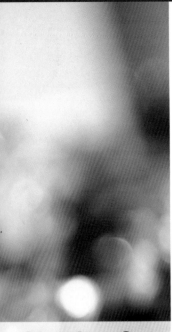

Lunches & light meals

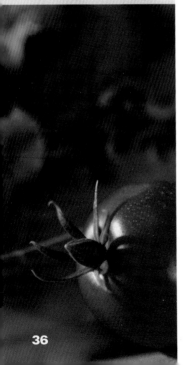

Mediterranean mixed salad

Here's a recipe that will bring back memories of hot summer days and balmy evenings on the beach anywhere in the Mediterranean. Wonderful ripe tomatoes, succulent and flavoursome sweet peppers and the coolness of cucumber add up to a feast of vitamins and anti-ageing free radical fighters.

Serves 4
Per serving

318 calories	19g fat
3g saturated fat	6g fibre

Ingredients
350g (12oz) frozen sweet corn
1 red pepper (diced)
1 yellow pepper (diced)
1 medium cucumber (peeled and diced)
150g (5oz) radishes (sliced)
1 sweet Spanish onion (finely chopped)
5 plum tomatoes (finely chopped)
110g (4oz) raisins
100ml (3.5fl oz) French dressing with herbs (see p47)

Method
1. Cook the sweet corn and leave to cool.
2. Put all the ingredients into a bowl with the raisins. Pour over the dressing and toss.

Watercress, chicory, onion, black grapes & alfalfa

Like all sprouted seeds, alfalfa sprouts are a rich source of nutrients including prebiotics. The chicory, onion and watercress also top up levels of prebiotics. Meanwhile, with all the phytochemicals in watercress, the natural sugars in grapes and plenty of vitamin C, this is a maximum-vitality dish.

Serves 4
Per serving

146 calories	4g fat
2g saturated fat	3g fibre

Ingredients
2 large bunches or bags watercress
3 heads chicory (leaves separated)
1 large Spanish onion (chopped)
400g (14oz) seedless black grapes (halved)
450g (1lb) alfalfa sprouts or bean sprouts
75ml (9fl oz) creamy dressing (see p46)

Method
1. Mix all the ingredients together then pour over the dressing and toss.

Tabbouleh

The mixture of bulghar wheat, cucumber and mint is what gives this dish its distinctly Middle Eastern flavour and large dose of prebiotics. A portion of this gives you well in excess of your daily requirement of vitamin C.

Serves 4
Per serving
486 calories   37g fat
5g saturated fat   3g fibre

Ingredients
110g (4oz) bulghar wheat
1 medium cucumber (diced)
1 large red onion (chopped)
4 large tomatoes (chopped)
6 large sprigs each mint and
    parsley (chopped)
150g (5oz) blueberries
200ml (7fl oz) standard
    French dressing with herbs
    (see p47)

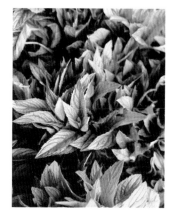

Method
1. Put the bulghar wheat into a bowl, cover with cold water and leave until swollen – about 30 mins.
2. Drain the bulghar wheat. Mix in the cucumber, onion, tomatoes, mint and parsley. Scatter the blueberries on top. Pour over the dressing.

Tomato, mozzarella & avocado salad

This is a far cry from the popular tricolore salad of 1970s Italian restaurants. The slices of red tomato, white mozzarella and green avocado are complemented by the nutritious dried fruits, vitamin C from the kiwi and an extremely high content of protective antioxidants. A salad to turn back your biological clock.

Serves 4
Per serving
318 calories   19g fat
5g saturated fat   8g fibre

Ingredients
175g (6oz) mixed dried fruits
    – dates, stoneless prunes,
    apricots, raisins etc.
    (snipped)
75ml French dressing with
    herbs (see p47)
4 large tomatoes (sliced)
2 kiwi fruit (sliced)
100g (12oz) mozzarella
    cheese (sliced)
1 avocado (sliced lengthwise)

Method
1. Soak all the fruits in freshly boiled water for 5 mins. Drain thoroughly and stir into the dressing.
2. Arrange the slices of tomato, mozzarella, kiwi fruit and avocado, in that order, on four plates. Pour over the fruit dressing and serve.

Beetroot, pink grapefruit, chicory & red onion salad

The visual appeal of these wonderful colours is enough to make you feel good before you even taste it. But when you add the benefits of beetroot, the heart-protective qualities from the grapefruit and the disease-fighting chemicals in onions, you really do have good health and prebiotics on a plate.

Serves 4
Per serving
84 calories   <1g fat
0g saturated fat   2g fibre

Ingredients
4 small, cooked beetroot
    (sliced)
2 pink grapefruit
    (divided into segments)
2 spears of chicory (sliced)
2 red onions (sliced)
1 quantity creamy dressing
    with yoghurt (see p46)

Method
1. Arrange the salad ingredients alternately around the sides of four plates or in a salad bowl. Pour over the dressing.

Cream of broccoli & brussels sprouts soup with almonds

This is one sure way to get youngsters to eat brussels and broccoli, although it's probably best to leave out the almonds for young children just in case of allergies. It's a cancer-protective soup as these vegetables are exceptionally rich in anti-cancer plant chemicals. The chickpeas supply the body with fermentable carbohydrates. Add a wholemeal roll and a glass of wine (adults only!) and you won't want much else.

Serves 4
Per serving
365 calories   28g fat
5g saturated fat   6.5g fibre

Ingredients
3tbsp extra virgin olive oil
1 onion (chopped)
1 clove garlic
1.2 litres (2 pints) basic stock (see p47)
1 bouquet garni
2 medium head broccoli (cut into florets)
350g (12oz) brussels sprouts (halved)
110g (4oz) ground almonds
150g canned chickpeas (drained)
100ml (10fl oz) single cream
4tbsp slivered almonds

Method
1. Heat the oil. Add the onion garlic, and sweat gently in the oil for 5 mins. Add the stock and bring to the boil.
2. Add the broccoli to the pan. Pick over the brussels sprouts and add to the pan. Add the bouquet garni and ground almonds.
3. Simmer gently for 10 mins, add the chickpeas, remove bouquet garni and simmer for another 5 minutes. Allow to cool a little before liquidising, in a food processor and return to pan.
4. Stir in the cream and heat through. Serve with the slivered almonds floating on top.

For a creamier but higher fat version of this recipe, add more cream (up to 300ml)

Salade Nicoise

This is a traditional recipe from the south of France. If you've ever eaten it under the Mediterranean sun, you'll only need one sniff of its distinctive aroma to transport you back to pavement cafés and happy memories. This dish contains lots of essential fatty acids and bone-building vitamin D from the fish, plus it's packed with carbohydrate, protein, vitamins A and C, iron and plenty of prebiotics from the artichoke.

Serves 4
Per serving
524 calories   39g fat
6g saturated fat   5g fibre

Ingredients
225g (8oz) waxy new potatoes like Jersey Royals
4 eggs
175g (6oz) French beans (trimmed)
1 large cos lettuce (separated)
2 x 160g (6oz) canned tuna in springwater (drained)
Half a cucumber (peeled)
2 large Jerusalem artichokes (sliced)
4 plum tomatoes (chopped)
100g can or jar anchovies (drained)
10 stoned black olives (halved)
150ml (5fl oz) standard French dressing with herbs (see p47)

Method
1. Boil potatoes until tender. Halve and leave to cool.
2. Semi hard-boil the eggs for 6 mins, rinse under cold running water to prevent discolouring. Peel and quarter when they're cool enough to handle.
3. Simmer the beans until just tender. Cut into 2.5cm (1in) sticks. Lay the lettuce leaves in a large bowl. Pile on the potatoes and beans.
4. Arrange on the beans. Add the cucumber and artichokes to the bowl. Cut into julienne strips and add to the bowl.
5. Pile the tomatoes on top. Add the quartered eggs. Arrange the artichokes on top of the eggs. Scatter the olives on top. Pour on the dressing.

Chilled cherry soup

A favourite from Eastern Europe, where luscious cherries grow in abundance. They're not only an extremely rich source of vitamin C, but also contain a group of naturally-occurring chemicals called bioflavonoids, which may help protect the inner walls of your veins and arteries. The sweetness of the wine adds to its taste.

Serves 4
Per serving
189 calories   <1g fat
0g saturated fat   2g fibre

Ingredients
800g (1lb 12 oz) fresh cherries (stoned weight)
200ml (7 fl oz) prune juice
200ml (7 fl oz) sweet white wine such as Sauternes
3tbsp runny honey
2tbsp arrowroot

Method
1. Put all but four of the cherries into a processor and whizz until smooth. Press firmly through a sieve to remove any remaining pieces of peel but to extract their juices.
2. Put the prune juice, white wine and honey into a saucepan. Heat gently until the honey is fully dissolved. Add the cherry pureé and heat gently.
3. Meanwhile, mix the arrowroot with a little water in a small bowl to make a smooth paste. Pour into the soup and continue heating very gently until the soup starts to thicken.
4. Take off the heat, leave to cool, then put into the fridge to chill. Halve the remaining four cherries, float on the soup and serve.

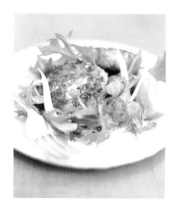

Tuna fishcakes

Fishcakes are a perennial family favourite and taste just as good hot or cold. Two make a substantial light meal; one makes an excellent starter. With the added nutritional value and cancer protection from the leafy green vegetables, you can turn this humble dish into a healthfest.

Serves 4
Per serving
319 calories   6g fat
2g saturated fat   5g fibre

Ingredients
200g (7oz) potatoes (peeled)
275g (10oz) green leafy vegetables eg kale, spring green, cabbage, spinach, pak choi etc (shredded)
6 spring onions (chopped)
2 x 160g (6oz) cans of tuna in springwater (drained and flaked)
3 eggs
6tbsp flour
Rapeseed oil for frying
1 iceberg lettuce (shredded)
1 quantity hot tomato salsa (see p47)

Method
1. Boil and roughly mash the potatoes. Steam until tender.
2. Tip the tuna into a large bowl. Add the onions. Stir in the potatoes and vegetable leaves and mix thoroughly.
3. Beat the eggs in a bowl. Tip the flour into another bowl. Mould the fish and potato mixture into eight flattened cakes. Dip each one first into the egg, then the flour.
4. Using sufficient oil to reach half way up the fish cakes, fry them in batches, over a medium heat, until golden – about 5 mins each side. Drain the finished cakes on a double layer of kitchen paper.
5. Divide the lettuce between four plates. Drizzle with some of the salsa. Put the fish cakes on top. Serve with the rest of the salsa on the side.

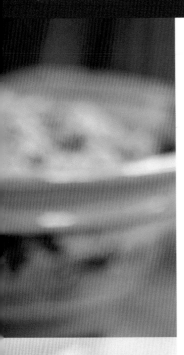

Dinners

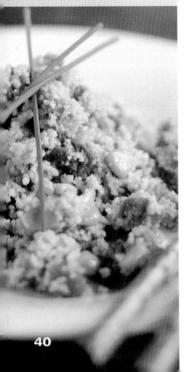

Risotto with peas & asparagus tips

Don't even think about risotto if you haven't got arborio rice and time. No other variety of rice works as well and you can't make good risotto in a hurry. Peas and asparagus add valuable prebiotics, and together with the spinach make this creamy, light risotto really nutritious. The bonus is the extra calcium from the mascarpone.

Serves 4
Per serving
411 calories   18g fat
4g saturated fat   7g fibre

Ingredients
4 plump spring onions
   (chopped into large sections)
3tbsp olive oil
225g (8oz) arborio rice
150g (6oz) frozen peas
12 asparagus tips
900ml (1 3/4pints) basic
   stock (see p47)
110g (4oz) baby spinach/rocket
3tbsp mascarpone cheese

Method
1. Heat the oil in a large saucepan and gently sauté the onions for 2 mins.
2. Add the rice and stir for 1 min. Mix in the peas and asparagus tips and add enough stock just to cover. Stir until the stock is almost absorbed.
3. Continue gradually adding the stock and stirring until the rice is tender.
4. Add the spinach or rocket and stir for 1 min. Stir in the mascarpone cheese.

Shrimp couscous with raisins

The mixture of couscous, raisins and shrimps with the spicy fish dressing provides the distinctive Middle Eastern flavour of this recipe. Quick and simple, this makes a delicious light meal for four or a starter for six.

Serves 4
Per serving
620 calories   20g fat
4g saturated fat   6g fibre

Ingredients
175g (6oz) raisins
350g (12oz) couscous
About 500ml (1 pint) basic
   stock (see p47)
225g (8oz) cooked, peeled
   shrimps
Half a large cucumber (cubed)
1 red pepper (cubed)
1 green pepper (cubed)
4 large plum tomatoes
   (chopped)
4 spring onions (chopped)
1 large carrot (grated)
1 courgette (grated)
100ml spicy dressing for fish
   (see p46)

Method
1. Put the raisins into freshly-boiled water for 1 min. Drain. Add to the couscous and cook according to packet instructions using basic stock instead of water – this usually takes about 20 mins. Stir in the shrimps when still warm.
2. Add the raw vegetables to the warm couscous mixture. Stir in the dressing. Serve while still warm, or cover with film and chill.

Braised duck with prunes

The combined flavours of duck, shallots, Armagnac and prunes are worthy of any Michelin star restaurant, but the recipe is simplicity itself. It has all the heart-protective benefits of garlic, shallots and red wine, lots of fibre, and huge amounts of beta-carotene. Add a simple salad for vitamin C and you'll have everything your body needs.

Serves 4
Per serving

483 calories	14g fat
3g saturated fat	10g fibre

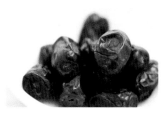

Ingredients
2tbsp extra virgin olive oil
4 duck breasts (skinless)
110g lean back bacon, diced
200g (7oz) shallots
3tbsp Armagnac
2tbsp flour
600ml (1 pint) red wine
10 stoned prunes
10 dried apricots
3 cloves garlic
1 bouquet garni

Method
1. Heat the oil in a frying pan and brown the duck breasts on both sides. Remove and keep warm.
2. Brown the bacon and shallots in the pan. Return the duck. Pour over the Armagnac and set alight. When the flames die down completely, stir in the flour and mix thoroughly.
3. Put into a casserole dish. Add half the wine to the frying pan, with the fruit, garlic and bouquet garni. Bring to the boil and pour in the rest of the wine.
4. Cook at 220C/425F/gas 7 for 20 mins.

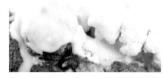

Broccoli & cauliflower cheese

The cancer-protective properties of broccoli and cauliflower are well documented and the lycopene from the tomatoes adds a huge prostate-protective boost for men and may help to reduce the risk of breast cancer for women. *(Cut out the Parmesan and reduce the amount of cheese sauce if you want to reduce the fat in this recipe)*

Serves 4
Per serving

417 calories	31g fat
13g saturated fat	4g fibre

Ingredients
1 large cauliflower (cut into florets)
2 large heads of broccoli (cut into florets)
2 small jars semi-dried tomatoes (drained and halved)
100g (7oz) strong Cheddar cheese (grated)
25g (2oz) unsalted butter
2tbsp flour
350ml (11/4 pints) semi-skimmed milk
4 large plum tomatoes (sliced)
2tbsp freshly grated Parmesan cheese

Method
1. Put the cauliflower and broccoli into a saucepan of boiling water, cook for 5 mins, drain and refresh under cold water. Arrange alternate florets in rows in a flat casserole dish.
2. Scatter the semi-dried tomatoes on the vegetables.
3. Heat the butter gently in a large frying pan. When melted, stir in the flour and cook for 2 mins, stirring constantly, until the mixture thickens. Gradually add the milk, again stirring continuously, and continue cooking until it forms a sauce. Add the grated cheese and stir until it's completely melted.
4. Pour the sauce over the vegetables. Arrange the plum tomatoes on top. Sprinkle with the Parmesan.
5. Bake at 220C/425F/gas 7 for 20 mins until the sauce is bubbling.

Steamed salmon with olive oil & vegetables

A brilliantly easy way to cook fish and the healthiest way to cook the vegetables. This produces a finished dish that's packed with essential nutrients and, thanks to the leeks, rich in prebiotics. Like all oily fish, the salmon provides heart, joint and brain-friendly essential fatty acids.

Serves 4
Per serving

472 calories	35g fat
8g saturated fat	7g fibre

Ingredients
2 small carrots (sliced lengthwise)
1 orange pepper (sliced)
4 spring onions (sliced lengthwise)
4 steaks of salmon
4tbsp extra virgin olive oil
Juice of 1 lemon
1 glass dry white wine
50g (2oz) unsalted butter
4 sprigs dill
Black pepper, freshly ground
700g (1lb 8oz) mixed green leafy vegetables – spinach, chard, cabbage, kale etc (chopped)
2 leeks (sliced)

Method
1. Cut four pieces of kitchen foil large enough to envelope each piece of fish comfortably. Put each fish steak into the middle of the foil. Divide the carrots, peppers and spring onions between them.
2. Pull up the sides and pour in the wine and lemon juice. Dot each parcel with butter, lay the dill on top, add a twist of freshly-ground black pepper and seal. Bake in the oven at 200C/400F/gas 6 for 20 mins.
3. Put all the vegetables into a steamer and cook until they're just tender but still have some bite – about 10 mins.
4. When the fish is cooked, pile the vegetables onto individual serving plates. Carefully open one end of each parcel and pour the juices over the vegetables. Lay the fish on the vegetables, with the carrot, pepper, spring onions and dill on top lengthwise)

Stuffed red peppers

These are wonderful to eat hot or cold. Red peppers are a nutritional feast on their own, but when you add the valuable antioxidants and other phytochemicals from the sweet corn, watercress, fibre from the brown rice and prebiotics from the onions, you've got an all round feast.

Serves 4
Per serving

320 calories	14g fat
5g saturated fat	6g fibre

Ingredients
110g (4oz) brown rice
1 large onion (chopped)
2tbsp extra virgin olive oil
200g (7oz) frozen sweet corn
1 bunch or bag watercress
4 large, flat bottomed red peppers (cut in half, de-seed and remove membrane)
8tbsp freshly grated Parmesan cheese
1 quantity hot tomato salsa (see p47)

Method
1. Cook the rice according to instructions on the packet. Sauté the onion gently in the oil until soft – about 5 mins.
2. Drain the cooked rice, pour into the onion mixture and stir until coated with the oil. Add the sweet corn and mix thoroughly.
3. Mix in the watercress leaves. Soak the peppers in boiling water for 5 mins. Remove and stand in a large baking or casserole dish.
4. Spoon the rice mixture into the pepper. Add 5tbsp of water to the dish. Cover with foil and bake at 180C/350F/gas 4 for 30 mins.
5. Remove the foil and sprinkle on the Parmesan cheese. Return to the oven for 10 mins.
6. Serve with the hot tomato salsa on the side. Sprinkle on the Parmesan cheese. Return to the oven for 10 mins.
7. Serve with the hot tomato salsa on the side.

Curried bean & root vegetable casserole

This is a perfect autumn or winter dish, and although it may look rather lengthy, it takes at most, half an hour to prepare and is the ideal dish for a slow cooker. Do all the preparation the night before, put into your slow cooker before you leave for work and when you open the door in the evening, you'll be greeted by mouth watering smells and a delicious dinner that's ready to eat. This is one meal that's exceptionally rich in prebiotics, thanks to the beans and the vegetables.

Serves 4
Per serving
278 calories   10g fat
1g saturated fat   6g fibre

Ingredients
1 large leek (sliced)
1 large onion (chopped)
3 cloves garlic (chopped)
3tbsp rapeseed oil
3tsp good curry powder or paste
1 swede (cubed)
1 large parsnip (cubed)
2 carrots (cubed)
1 medium sweet potato (cubed)
About 700ml (1 1/4pints) basic stock (see p47)
400g can chopped tomatoes
3tbsp tomato pureé
1 400g can broad beans (drained)

Method
1. In a large saucepan, heat the oil and sweat the leek, onion and garlic, stirring continuously, for 3 mins.
2. Tip in the curry powder or paste, stir until it coats the vegetables and cook for another 2 mins.
3. Add the root vegetables to the pan and stir to coat thoroughly. Add the stock, chopped tomatoes and tomato pureé and bring to the boil.
4. Cover and simmer for 45 mins. Add the broad beans. to the pan. Continue to simmer until beans and vegetable are all tender – about 10-15 mins.

Vegetarian nutty bake

This is nut roast with attitude. This a health-plus recipe which will be enjoyed as much by committed carnivores as it will by the veggies. Everything you need and lots of prebiotics.

Serves 4
Per serving
200 calories   6g fat
3.5g saturated fat 2.7g fibre

Ingredients
25g (3oz) unsalted butter *(you may add more butter here, but the fat content of the recipe will be raised)*
1 onion (chopped)
2 cloves garlic (chopped)
350g (12oz) mixed root vegetables (diced)
1 leek (trimmed and sliced)
2 courgettes
200g (7oz) chestnut mushrooms (sliced)
50g (2oz) wholemeal flour
300ml (1/2 pint) basic stock (see p47)
4tbsp tomato pureé
100g (4oz) ready-to-eat prunes
2 large sprigs of curly parsley (chopped)
75g (3oz) porridge oats
75g (3oz) crushed mixed nuts

Method
1. Melt 20g (2oz) of the butter in a large frying pan. Add the onion and garlic and sweat gently in the butter until soft – about 5 mins.
2. Add the root vegetables to the pan and continue cooking gently for another 10 mins.
3. Add the leeks and mushrooms to the pan and cook for 1 min.
4. Stir in the flour and cook for 1 min, stirring continuously. Pour in the stock, tomato pureé and prunes and stir until thickened.
5. Add the parsley to the mixture. Season with freshly ground black pepper. Pour the mixture into an oven-proof dish.
6. Rub the remaining butter into the oats and nuts. Scatter onto the dish and bake at for 30 mins at 180C/350F/gas 4.

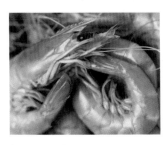

Prawns & vegetable stir fry

The way people eat in the Far East often holds the secret to their good health. In this part of the world, women have less breast cancer, hardly any osteoporosis and there's not even a word for menopausal hot flushes. Heart disease, high blood pressure and bowel cancer are comparatively rare. This great dish is a typical example of the type of meal served in the East. It includes prebiotics from the onion, peas and beansprouts.

Serves 4
Per serving

234 calories	16g fat
<1g saturated fat	9g fibre

Ingredients
1tbsp light soy sauce
1tbsp sherry vinegar
Half a tsp Tabasco sauce
1tbsp sesame oil
1tsp runny honey
5 fat spring onions
   (trimmed and sliced)
2 medium carrots
   (peeled and sliced)
1 medium head broccoli
   (cut into florets)
110g (4oz) oyster mushrooms
   (sliced)
2 medium heads pak choi
   (trimmed)
1.5cm (half inch) fresh ginger
   root (peeled and grated)
150g (6oz) mange tout (snipped)
2tbsp rapeseed oil
8 raw king tiger prawns,
   shells still on
450g (1lb) fresh beansprouts
4tbsp sesame seeds

Method
1. Whisk together the soy sauce, sherry vinegar, Tabasco sauce, sesame oil and honey and set aside.
2. Heat the rapeseed oil in a wok or large, deep-sided frying pan. Add the carrots, mushrooms, broccoli and ginger and stir-fry, stirring continuously, for 3 mins.
3. Add the spring onions, pak choi and mange tout and continue cooking for 1 min. Add the prawns and cook for 4 mins until they start to change colour.
4. Add the beansprouts and cook for 1 min. Add the soy sauce mixture and 3tbsp water and cook gently until the vegetables are tender – about 4 mins.
5. Meanwhile, dry fry the sesame seeds in a separate pan. Serve the stir fry with the sesame seeds scattered on top.

Mango chicken with raisins & walnuts

This dish offers a taste of the Pacific rim, as the exotic flavours of mango are combined with simple roast chicken. The monounsaturated fat in the walnuts provide additional heart protection.

Serves 4
Per serving

506 calories	40g fat
4g saturated fat	6g fibre

Ingredients
1 small, cold, roast chicken
   (skinned & chopped)
2 ripe mangoes (cubed)
4 large spring onions (sliced)
110g (4oz) raisins
Juice of 2 limes
100ml (31/2fl oz) extra-virgin
   olive oil
6tsp mayonnaise
50g (2oz) walnuts (chopped)
200g (7oz) rocket

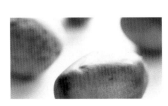

Method
1. Mix the chicken, mangoes and spring onions with the raisins, lime juice, oil and mayonnaise
2. Stir all the ingredients together.

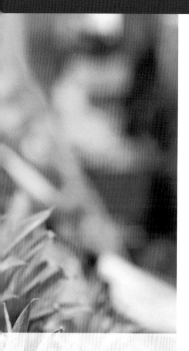

Desserts

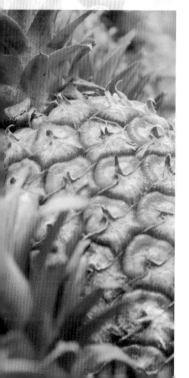

Plums roasted in red wine & cranberry Juice

This is a very simple dessert with a variety of health benefits. The cranberry juice may help relieve and prevent cystitis, the fresh mint may help digestion, the red wine is good for your heart and the plums provide fibre, vitamins and minerals.

Serves 4
Per serving
298 calories   10g fat
7g saturated fat   6g fibre

Ingredients
8 plump red plums (halved & de-stoned)
50g (2oz) unsalted butter
450ml (three-quarters of a pint) mixed red wine and cranberry juice
4 large sprigs mint (chopped)
4tbsp brown caster sugar

Method
1. Rub the bottom of a shallow casserole pan with some of the butter. Lay the plums on top, cut side down.
2. Sprinkle the mint leaves over the plums and dot over the remaining butter. Dust with the the sugar and pour on cranberry juice and red wine mixture.
3. Roast at 180C/350F/ gas 4 for 20 mins.

Spicy fruit kebabs with pineapple, mango, pawpaw & cinnamon

These simple fruit kebabs are quick, fun and healthy and you can cook them under the grill or on the barbecue when the weather's good.

Serves 4
Per serving
286 calories   <1g fat
0g saturated fat   4g fibre

Ingredients
1 medium pineapple
1 large mango, not too ripe
1 large pawpaw, not too ripe
2 bananas
125ml (4fl oz) runny honey
Half a tsp cinnamon

Method
1. Cut all the fruit into bite size pieces and thread onto skewers.
2. Drizzle the kebabs with honey, sprinkle with ground cinnamon. Cook under hot grill or on the barbecue in a foil lined pan for around 5 mins. Enjoy.

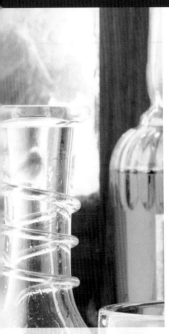

Sauces, dips & dressings

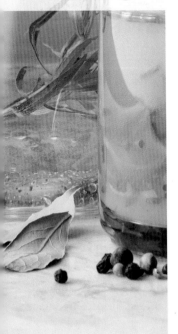

Spicy dressing

Perfect with seafood salad, or any type of fish salad using tuna, cod, salmon, trout or mackerel

Provides about 370g
Per 100g
590 calories   63g fat
7g saturated fat   <1g fibre

Ingredients
125ml (4fl oz) olive oil
125ml (4fl oz) walnut oil
2 small red chillies
   (de-seeded and chopped)
3 large spring onions (sliced)
1 clove garlic (chopped)
2.5cm (1in) fresh ginger
   (grated)

Method
1. Mix all the ingredients together and leave for an hour in the fridge for the flavours to combine. Unused dressing can be refrigerated in an airtight container for up to ten days

Creamy dressing with yoghurt

This cool, green dressing goes well with cold new potatoes, a mixed green salad or cold fresh salmon. Use sparingly especially if trying to reduce or manage your body weight.

Provides about 810g
Per 100g
64 calories   4g fat
<1g saturated fat <1g fibre

Ingredients
Half a cucumber (chopped)
1 sweet Spanish onion
   (chopped)
1 large green pepper (diced)
2 cloves garlic (chopped)
3tbsp olive oil
1 x 240 ml carton of natural,
   bio-yoghurt

Method
1. Mix yoghurt and olive oil together. Blend together with the vegetables for 1 min.

Yoghurt sauce

Wonderful served with hot or cold desserts. Provides vitamin C and all the digestive benefits of mint.

Provides about 470g
Per 100g
62 calories   <1g fat
<1g saturated fat 3g fibre

Ingredients
150g (5oz) blackcurrants
1 lemon (grated zest)
1 large sprig mint (chopped)
2tbsp honey
Half a tsp ground cinnamon
250ml (9fl oz) natural, live
   bio-yoghurt

Method
1. Simmer the blackcurrants gently in water for 5 – 10 mins until just tender. Push thoroughly through a fine sieve to remove the pips. Leave the pureé to cool completely.
2. Mix the lemon zest, honey, cinnamon and mint into the yogurt. When the blackcurrants are cold, stir them thoroughly into the yogurt mixture.

Standard french dressing

Despite the enormous influence of Mediterranean and oriental cooking on TV shows, getting a decent salad is still a comparative rarity and a true delight when you do. The secret is in the preparation and the dressing. Wash all salad well and dry thoroughly. Invest in a salad spinner, as even good quality dressings won't coat the surface of wet leaves. This dressing will go with any type of salad and will keep in an air-tight jar for at least a week – but don't put it in the fridge because it will solidify. Use sparingly (approx 20g per person), especially if you are trying to reduce or manage your body weight.

Provides about 350g
Per 100g
600 calories   66g fat
9g saturated fat   <1g fibre

Ingredients
250ml (9fl oz) extra virgin
  olive oil
175ml (6fl oz) herb vinegar
2tsp mild mustard
1 pinch of sea salt
3 generous twists black
  pepper
3tbsp chopped mixed
  herbs eg flat-leaf parsley,
  tarragon, marjoram, chervil
  and oregano

Method
1. Throw all the ingredients into a bowl, apart from the fresh herbs, and whisk until thickened.
2. Stir in the fresh herbs.

Hot tomato salsa

This extra hot and spicy salsa is ideal as a dip or accompaniment to hot or cold dishes.

Provides about 500g
Per 100g
26 calories   <1g fat
0g saturated fat   1g fibre

Ingredients
1 medium red onion
  (chopped finely)
3 large tomatoes
  (peeled and chopped)
2 large red chillies
  (de-seeded and chopped)
4tbsp tomato pureé
3 sprigs of fresh coriander
  (chopped)

Method
1. Mix all the ingredients together and leave to chill in the fridge for an hour.

Basic stock

With instant stock cubes and 'fresh' stock on the supermarket shelves, the art of stock-making is disappearing fast. That's a great shame as none of the commercially-prepared varieties taste as good as your own and they're usually loaded with salt. It's easy to make your own stock – and it freezes well, too. Simply, turn it into ice cubes, which can then be used from frozen to enhance stews, casserole, sauces and soups. This is one traditional kitchen skill that handsomely repays such a small investment in time and effort.

Provides about 1450g
Per 100g
24 calories   <1g fat
0g saturated fat   2.5g fibre

Ingredients
2 large onions
2 sticks celery with their leaves
4 large carrots (trimmed)
4 leeks (trimmed)
3 tomatoes (quartered)
2 stems thyme
1 large sprig rosemary
2 bay leaves
6 peppercorns

Method
1. Peel and slice one onion. Leave the other whole and unpeeled as the skin will give extra colour to the stock.
2. Put all the ingredients into a large saucepan with about 4 litres of water (if you have a pasta or asparagus pan with an inside sieve, that would be ideal). Simmer gently without a lid for two hours till reduced by at least one third.
3. Pour through a colander and drain into another pot, then tip the vegetables into a fine sieve and press with a wooden spoon to extract as much liquid as possible.

Exercises for a healthy digestive system

By Nicki Waterman

Exercise can play an important part in keeping the digestive system healthy. But as well as helping to exercise the muscles of the digestive tract and helping to control our weight, exercise also has the added benefit of helping to reduce stress.

Our digestive tract is ringed with muscles that contract to help move food through. Like other muscles in our bodies, these muscles are stimulated by exercise. And by exercising regularly you will keep the bowel muscles contracting at a healthy rate.

Fortunately, you don't need to become a gym fanatic or cross country champion to gain the benefits of regular exercise. Simply being more active in your daily life is a good starting point.

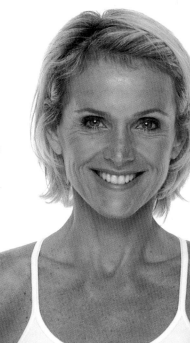

Try incorporating some of these activities into your routine...

- Leave the car at home for short distances and walk to the shops, school, pub or post office.
- Don't wait for ages to park your car next to the supermarket entrance – walking that bit further won't do you any harm.
- Ban all lifts and escalators and use the stairs instead
- Plug the phone in upstairs so that every time it rings you have to climb the stairs (and then come down them again)
- Don't pile clutter up at the bottom of the stairs – take items upstairs individually
- Stop shopping online and instead return to walking around your favourite shopping centres
- Browse around the shops at lunchtime instead of reading a magazine in the office.

It is also important to do some form of activity that increases your heart rate and gets you breathing heavily. While aerobic activities such as running, cycling, swimming and aerobics classes can all achieve this, brisk walking will also do the job.

For good health, experts recommend we take 10,000 steps every day. However, most of us don't even come close to this. Walking is a great form of exercise that can be accomplished by almost anyone.

Top tips to better walking

1. Plan ahead. Try using an iPod or other MP3 player to add entertainment to your walk. Music will probably make you want to walk faster and you may find you even want to walk for longer

2. Set some realistic goals – if you've been sedentary for a long time, you should start out slowly and aim for short distances

3. Pay attention to your posture – stand up straight, put your shoulders back, and take long strides

4. Don't worry about how far you walk. The length of time you walk for is more important than the distance. Faster and further will come later.

5. Increase the length of your sessions over time – aim for a five minute increase each time you walk

6. Once you can comfortably walk for 45 minutes a day, start to work on your distance and increase the difficulty of the walk, for example, start to incorporate hills into your walk

7. Aim to walk a minimum of four times a week. If you can, incorporate a walk into your daily routine. On weekends or holidays, try to increase your walking time to an hour or more

8. You'll get the most out of your exercise if you walk to your target heart rate. To do this, subtract your age from 220 to find your maximum heart rate. Then, multiply that number by 0.8 to get your target heart rate. For example, if you are 40 years old, your maximum heart rate is 180. Your target heart rate is 144.

9. Wear proper footwear – sandals, flip-flops and even fashion 'sports' shoes don't support the various muscles, tendons and joints in your foot and can therefore cause strain and injury.

10. Don't carry weights when you walk – any extra weight will throw your gait out of balance and is the leading cause of conditions that need orthopedic surgery.

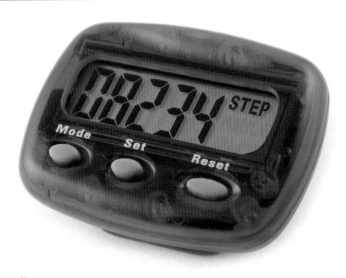

Using a pedometer to get fit

Digital pedometers clip onto your belt and record not only your steps (based on body movement) but will convert those steps to miles. Some even tell the time and estimate the calories you've burned based on your body weight. Pedometers work well for people who simply don't have or take time to walk consistently as a form of exercise. By tracking the number of steps you take each day simply doing your regular daily activities, you may find that you're getting in plenty of exercise. Some experts recommend 10,000 steps a day.

In normal daily activity, adults cover about 2-3 miles (2,000 steps/ mile). To make walking a beneficial activity, you would need to come up with at least another 4,000 steps in a day. You can find ways to add steps here and there, such as walking further from car parks, taking stairs instead of escalators and lifts, walking the long way to get somewhere in your office building, walking your children to school, or planning a short walk around the block as a break.

Be kind to yourself - Yoga & Pilates

Some digestive disorders such as constipation may be brought on by, or made worse by stress. Finding a leisure activity that focuses on breathing, body control and relaxation will help you to de-stress. Most gyms now offer classes in yoga, pilates and stretching: your local paper or library should be able to point you in the right direction.

Also, when we breathe properly more oxygen is taken into our lungs - and consequently into our blood - to help the process of digestion.

Fortunately you don't have to spend hours in a class – just 10 minutes at home each day will help to relax and de-stress your digestive system. Try these simple stretching exercises which aid digestion by freeing the rib-cage and allowing for improved breathing. Stretching also helps to slow heartbeat, strengthen the lower back and remove pressure from the lumbar region. Finally, it increases flexibility and strengthens and develops the hamstrings.

1. The standing forward bend

a. Stand in the centre of your mat, with your hands in prayer position. Jump your feet wide apart. Keep the outside of your feet parallel with each other while lifting your arches, pulling up with the thighs and tucking the tail bone under. Place your hands on your hips and feel the extension up out of the waist.

b. Inhale. As you exhale bend at the hips extend forward, continue lifting out of the hips keeping your legs strong and your base nice and firm, looking forward. Keep the extension on the stomach, which will help keep your back flat protecting it. Take a few breaths.

c. Now take your hands to the floor extending from the lower abdomen to the breastbone and through the spine.

d. If you can't keep your spine straight put your hands on your knees and keep working down your legs, working with your body, not against it. Lift your sitting bones to the ceiling. Draw your shoulders down your back so you can extend the neck with ease. Remember - keep the arches high.

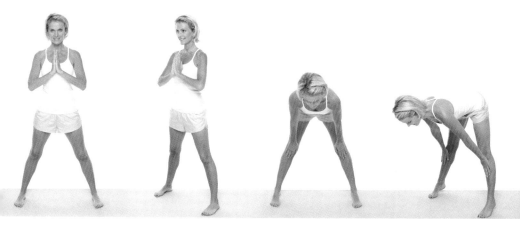

2. Energising breath & arm toner

Low energy levels and tiredness are very ageing, so keep topping up your energy with this movement. It's a lovely deep breathing exercise to start your day.

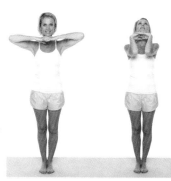

Stand straight with feet together and interlock your hands under your chin. Inhale deeply for a count of five through your nose, lifting your elbows. Drop your head back slightly as you exhale through your mouth, drawing your elbows together. Bring your head up again, draw your elbows up and repeat five times

3. Upwards stretch, forward & backward bend & leg lengthener

This movement releases tension from the whole body, gently stretches and tones the spine, tones the muscles of the legs, firming the back of the thigh area, and is marvellous for the skin and hair due to the extra blood stimulated to the head and neck.

Stand very straight with your feet a little apart. Inhale and slowly lift your arms, stretching them above your head. Exhale as you move forward into your maximum forward stretch, without bending your knees – until your chin is on your knees. Hold for 5 seconds, breathing normally, and inhale as you stretch back to forward position and exhale again, lowering your arms. Repeat.

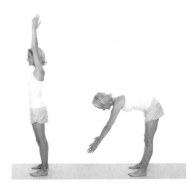

4. Chest expansion & bust booster

Use this movement to relax the muscles at the back of the shoulders and get rid of the proverbial 'pain in the neck'.

Stand straight and interlock your arms behind your back, keeping elbows straight. Inhale and raise your arms as high as possible and hold for a count of five. Exhale and gently lower your head towards the floor, continuing to lift the arms. Hold for five seconds, breathing normally. Inhale and return to a standing position, keeping the arms held up behind your back. Then relax the upper body backward, pulling your arms down under your bottom. Inhale and come up. Lower your arms and you should experience a lovely warm glow as the shoulders and neck muscles relax. Repeat five times.

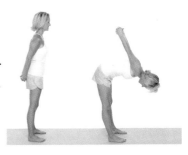

5. Half moon posture & waist whittler

This brilliant exercise corrects posture, whittles the waistline, firms the back of the thighs and is excellent for spine flexibility.

Stand straight with your feet together and your back totally straight. Inhale and lift your arms above your head, elbows slightly bent; and stretch upwards. Exhale as you slowly move your torso to the right, pushing the hips to the left, without moving your feet. Hold for five seconds. Inhale as you return to an upright position and stretch up. Repeat, moving to the left this time, then do a forward bend and backward bend in turn, keeping the legs straight.

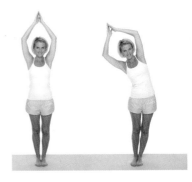

6. Triangle & tummy toner

This exercise will help keep the lower back agile. It is also great for the flexibility of your hips, for toning the back of the thighs and reducing flab around the waist and hips.

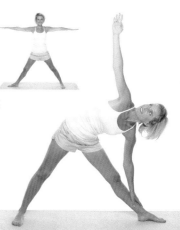

Stand straight and place the legs about four feet apart, placing the right foot out at 90-degrees and the left foot facing forwards. Place your arms straight out at the sides. Reach to your right. Inhale, and as you exhale keep legs straight and clasp the right leg with your right hand. (If possible, place the hand flat on the floor with the little finger by the big toe). Lift the left arm up straight and turn your head to look at the ceiling, pulling the shoulder back so your fingertips point to the ceiling. Hold for five seconds, inhale and return to standing. Repeat on the other side. Do whole exercise twice.

7. Wide angled forward & backward stretch & bottom toner

The backward stretch is excellent if you are sitting at a desk all day, and it really helps the lungs and chest. It's also good for toning and firming the backs of the legs and buttocks.

Stand with your legs about four feet apart and stretch up as you inhale. Exhale. Keeping your head up, your back flat and your legs straight, allow your body to move carefully forward. Slip your hands behind your legs, and as you exhale, draw your head in towards your knees. Relax and hold the position for five seconds, breathing normally. Lifting just your head, start to inhale as you gently come up into standing position. With a full lung, gently place the thumbs in front of your waistline and fingers at the back, and gently relax the body backwards. Exhale and hold for 5 seconds, breathing normally. Inhale as you return to a standing position, exhale and relax. Repeat.

Warm up. Always begin with at least 5 minutes of walking, stair climbing or other low-intensity activity, raising the body temperature by 5 to 10 degrees. A warmed muscle both contracts more forcefully and relaxes more quickly, and the probability of overstretching a muscle and causing injury is far less.

Use the rules of thumb. Stretching should result in tension in the muscles but not pain. If it hurts, lessen the stress until it stops. Always keep in mind this isn't about pushing your body to the limit, it is about gentle stretching. Also, never bounce in the pose. It can cause injury by over stretching warmed muscles. Ease into the stretch gently.

Digestive Yoga

The following poses have been long used within the practices of yoga specifically to aid digestion:

1. Yogasana

a. Sit as in easy pose. Clasp hands behind the back, Straighten arms as much as possible, thus pulling shoulders back "soldier" fashion.

b. Begin to push the hands upwards behind you, at the same time allowing the head to bend forward towards the ground.

c. Do not force the pose. Do not worry if at first you hardly bend forward at all. Begin by holding the pose for 15 seconds, working up to one minute.

Aims & results:

To stretch spine, shoulders, neck, knees and hips; to massage the nerves of the spine, and the organs in the abdomen. Yoga experts claim this move can aid poor posture and indigestion.

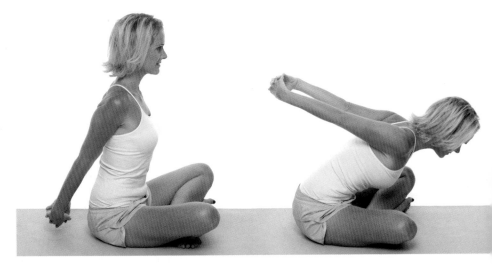

2. Tortoise

a. Sit on floor with knees drawn up slightly, feet and knees wide apart.

b. Put the arms in between the legs taking hold of the ankles.

c. Droop forward as far as you can between knees. Then begin to pull slightly, bringing head towards the ground.

d. Eventually head will touch the ground. Arms can then be extended backwards, making the body look likes tortoise.

Aims and results:

Carries on stretching the body forward, slimming waist and strengthening stomach.
Yoga experts claim this move prevents constipation, coldness, poor circulation, bad digestion and breath odour.

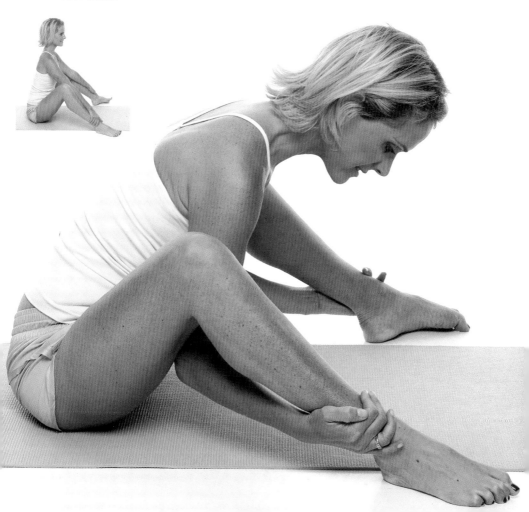

WEEK COMMENCING ....|........	BREAKFAST	LUNCH	DINNER	SNACKS	WATER (GLASSES)
EXAMPLE DAY	2 slices wholegrain toast with peanut butter 1 banana	three bean salad 1 pear	pea and asparagus risotto	2 oatcakes with avocado and low fat cream cheese	6
MONDAY					
TUESDAY					
WEDNESDAY					
THURSDAY					
FRIDAY					
SATURDAY					
SUNDAY					

PROBIOTIC DRINK	PREBIOTICS IN DIET	HOURS OF SLEEP	HOURS OF TV	HOURS OF EXERCISE	ENERGY LEVEL 1 = LOW 10 = HIGH
Yakult	banana asparagus spring onions chickpeas kidney beans oats	6	3	3o mins	7

Contacts & organisations

Please contact Yakult for free information on digestive
health and probiotics.

UK

Write to	Yakult FREEPOST
Log on to	www.yakult.co.uk
Telephone	0845 769 7069

ROI

Write to	Yakult Ireland
	Suite 117
	52 Broomhill Rd.
	Tallaght, Dublin 24
Log on to	www.yakult.ie
Telephone	1890 946 221

**To order an additional copy of this booklet or to share your
experience of The Inside Out Diet, please visit the dedicated
website, www.insideoutdiet.co.uk**

Below is a list of suggested websites for further information.

The listed organisations do not necessarily endorse the The Inside Out Diet or any commercial products, and neither Yakult nor The Inside Out Diet authors are responsible for the content of any listed sites. *All links are correct at time of going to press.*

Digestive health support organisations

Core (corecharity.org.uk)
IBS Network (ibsnetwork.org.uk)
The National Association for Colitis and Crohn's Disease (NACC) (nacc.org.uk)
The Colostomy Association (colostomyassociation.org.uk)
Coeliac UK (coeliac.org.uk)
InContact (incontact.org)

Health sites

NHS Direct (nhsdirect.nhs.uk)
Net Doctor (netdoctor.co.uk)
(netdoctor.co.uk/digestive)
What Really Works (whatreallyworks.co.uk)
Directgov (direct.gov.uk/HealthAndWellBeing)
Patient UK (patient.co.uk)
BUPA (bupa.co.uk/health_information)
iVillage (ivillage.co.uk/health)
BBC Health (bbc.co.uk/health)
Health Space (healthspace.nhs.uk)
Saga Health (saga.co.uk/health)
Gut Week (gutweek.org.uk)

Diet/nutrition

FSA (food.gov.uk)
FSA Eat Well (eatwell.gov.uk)
NHS 5 a Day (5aday.nhs.uk)
BNF (nutrition.org.uk)
British Dietetic Association Weightwise (bdaweightwise.com)
National Obesity Forum (nationalobesityforum.org)

Exercise/sport

Net Fit (netfit.co.uk)
Sport England (sportengland.org)
UK Sport (uksport.gov.uk)
Active Places (activeplaces.com)
Culture, Media & Sport dept (culture.gov.uk)
The Ramblers' Association (ramblers.org.uk)
BBC Gardening (bbc.co.uk/gardening/)
Royal Horticultural Society (rhs.org.uk)
Yoga UK (yogauk.com)
British Wheel of Yoga (bwy.org.uk)
Pilates Foundation (pilatesfoundation.com)
Walking the Way to Health (whi.org.uk)
Directgov (direct.gov.uk/leisureandrecreation)

Mental/cultural health/stress management

Sleep Council (sleepcouncil.com)
24 Hour Museum (24hourmuseum.org.uk)
MIND (mind.org.uk)
HSE Stress section (HSE.gov.uk/stress)

Travel

Travel Health (travelhealth.co.uk)

Smoking

Giving Up Smoking (givingupsmoking.co.uk)

Alcohol

Alcohol Concern (alcoholconcern.org.uk)
Alcoholics Anonymous (alcoholics-anonymous.org.uk)

Height (Feet and Inches)

	5'0"	5'1"	5'2"	5'3"	5'4"	5'5"	5'6"	5'7"	5'8"	5'9"	5'10"	5'11"	6'0"	6'1"	6'2"	6'3"	6'4"	
45	20	19	18	18	17	17	16	16	15	15	14	14	14	13	13	12	12	7st1lb
47	21	20	19	19	18	17	17	16	16	16	15	15	14	14	13	13	13	7st5lb
50	21	21	20	19	19	18	18	17	17	16	16	15	15	15	14	14	13	7st9lb
52	22	22	21	20	20	19	19	18	17	17	17	16	16	15	15	14	14	8st2lb
54	23	23	22	21	21	20	19	19	18	18	17	17	16	16	15	15	15	8st6lb
57	24	24	23	22	21	21	20	20	19	18	18	17	17	16	16	16	15	8st9lb
59	25	25	24	23	22	22	21	20	20	19	19	18	18	17	17	16	16	9st3lb
61	26	26	25	24	23	22	22	21	21	20	19	19	18	18	17	17	16	9st6lb
63	27	26	26	25	24	23	23	22	21	21	20	20	19	18	18	17	17	10st
66	28	27	27	26	25	24	23	23	22	21	21	20	20	19	19	18	18	10st4lb
68	29	28	27	27	26	25	24	23	23	22	22	21	20	20	19	19	18	10st7lb
70	30	29	28	27	27	26	25	24	24	23	22	22	21	20	20	19	19	11st1lb
72	31	30	29	28	27	27	26	25	24	24	23	22	22	21	21	20	19	11st4lb
75	32	31	30	29	28	27	27	26	25	24	24	23	22	22	21	21	20	11st8lb
77	33	32	31	30	29	28	27	27	26	25	24	24	23	22	22	21	21	12st1lb
79	34	33	32	31	30	29	28	27	27	26	25	24	24	23	22	22	21	12st5lb
82	35	34	33	32	31	30	29	28	27	27	26	25	24	24	23	22	22	12st9lb
84	36	35	34	33	32	31	30	29	28	27	27	26	25	24	24	23	23	13st2lb
86	37	36	35	34	33	32	31	30	29	28	27	26	26	25	24	24	23	13st6lb
88	38	37	36	35	33	32	31	31	30	29	28	27	26	26	25	24	24	13st9lb
91	39	38	37	35	34	33	32	31	30	30	29	28	27	26	26	25	24	14st3lb
93	40	39	37	36	35	34	33	32	31	30	29	29	28	27	26	26	25	14st6lb
95	41	40	38	37	36	35	34	33	32	31	30	29	28	28	27	26	26	15st
98	42	41	39	38	37	36	35	34	33	32	31	30	29	28	28	27	26	15st4lb
100	43	42	40	39	38	37	36	34	33	32	32	31	30	29	28	27	27	15st7lb
102	44	43	41	40	39	37	36	35	34	33	32	31	31	30	29	28	27	16st1lb
104	45	43	42	41	39	38	37	36	35	34	33	32	31	30	30	29	28	16st4lb
107	46	44	43	42	40	39	38	37	36	35	34	33	32	31	30	29	29	16st8lb
109	47	45	44	43	41	40	39	38	36	35	34	33	33	32	31	30	29	17st1lb
111	48	46	45	43	42	41	40	38	37	36	35	34	33	32	31	31	30	17st5lb
114	49	47	46	44	43	42	40	39	38	37	36	35	34	33	32	31	30	17st9lb

Weight (Kilograms) — Weight (Stone and Pounds)

150   152.5   155   157.5   160   162.5   165   167.5   170   172.5   175   177.5   180   182.5   185   187.5   190

Height (Centimetres)

 Underweight

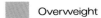 Weight appropriate

 Overweight

Obese

- A BMI of less than 18.5 (women) and 20 (men) indicates you are underweight. You may need to gain weight.
- A BMI of 18.5 to 24.9 (women) and 20 (men) to 24.9 indicates you are a healthy weight and should aim to stay that way.
- A BMI of 25 to 29.9 means you are overweight. It's a good idea to lose weight for your health, or at least aim to prevent further weight gain.
- A BMI of more than 30 means you are obese and putting your health at risk. Losing weight will improve your health.